LOOKING TO LOSE WEIGHT?

DUMP YOUR TRAINER

THE ONLY THING THEY'LL REDUCE IS YOUR WALLET!

by

Ashley Marriott, Certified Personal Trainer

and

Marc L. Paulsen, M.D.

Looking To Lose Weight?

Dump Your Trainer

The only thing they'll reduce is your wallet!

By: Ashley Marriott, Certified Personal Trainer and Marc Paulsen, M.D.

www.DumpYourTrainer.com

Artwork by Shawn Encarnacion

Library of Congress Control Number: 2007908759
Publisher: BookSurge Publishing
North Charleston, South Carolina

ISBN 1-4196-8023-4

Table of Contents

iv

Foreword

by
Marc L. Paulsen, M.D.

Over the last several years, personal training programs have exploded in popularity. Hardly a day goes by in which some talk show like *Oprah* isn't espousing the achievements of this or that "trainer to the stars." Tabloid news shows are constantly publicizing the miracles of some new "celebrity trainer." Television shows like *The Biggest Loser* attract huge ratings, but could be misleading the public in terms of expectations. Go into practically any fitness club these days and the walls are lined with photos of its team of young, attractive trainers. In some select fitness studios I've belonged to, if you didn't have a trainer you felt like a pariah.

Personal training is big business. The average cost per training session runs fifty to one hundred dollars and lasts 50–60 minutes. On average, clients book trainers three to five times per week. Thousands of facilities employ a multitude of trainers to service a growing number of hopeful clients. Add it all up and it's big, big money.

So, one may ask, with all this "fitness" going on, why is it that the American public is actually getting fatter? Obesity is increasingly a major health problem in this country, and diet books continue to be some of the top-selling books every year. But sadly, most people are still confused or clueless when it comes to knowing how to lose weight or find time to fit an exercise program into their daily routine.

Out of frustration, and induced by media hype and misinformation, often people will hire a personal trainer when they sign up at a health club or gym. But after weeks or months of making no progress, most of these once hopeful health seekers fall back into the same old routine of unhealthy eating and limited physical activity… and the cycle continues.

Ironically, because a typical trainer program focuses on muscle building instead of calorie burning through aerobic exercise and conditioning, people can be lulled into a false sense of accomplishment. Many trainer clients think that since they've worked out with a trainer they've burned a significant number of calories and can justify certain indulgences, such as a plate of cheese nachos, a pizza, or a hot fudge sundae.

The information in this book is presented as simply, enjoyably, and provocatively as possible. The main goal of this collaborative work is to steer people away from wasting their time and money on the fad of personal training, and to provide the essential basics of fitness and weight loss to empower the reader to take control of their own overall health. There are numerous medical, dietary, and other publications dealing with nutrition and the science of weight loss. If the reader has the inclination and time, we certainly encourage him or her to learn as much as possible. However, it is our assumption that in today's fast paced world that many don't have the time for this, and would benefit from a simple, straightforward guide to achieving their weight loss and health improvement goals. As you will learn in the following pages, just sitting around and reading burns only 50–80 calories per hour while aerobic exercise will burn 400–800 calories per hour, improve your cardiovascular health, and help you feel much better about your appearance.

A brief note on formatting

The book is largely a cooperative work by Ashley Marriott and Marc Paulsen, M.D. In some areas where a particular author wishes to emphasize her/his personal perspective an image will appear in the section or next to a note *in italics* representing

either Ashley's view or that of Doctor Paulsen .

Introduction

Sure, they're handsome/pretty, young, and toned. That's why the gyms hire them. But you don't need them, they're expensive, and they'll only get in the way of your losing weight. Why? Because most Personal Trainers will only waste your limited time doing the kind of exercises that burn very few calories, and don't increase your aerobic conditioning or improve your cardiovascular health. In fact, their exercise programs will increase your appetite so that you may end up consuming more calories than you actually expend – which means you may GAIN weight instead of losing it.

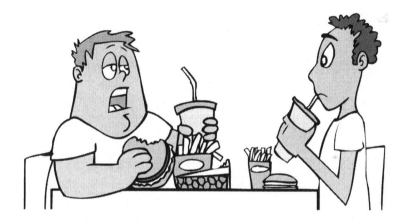

"I had a great workout with my trainer today. Ten minutes of squats, lunges, and weight training, along with forty minutes of trying to get her phone number. I even got my heart rate up to one-sixty when she bent over to get her iPhone."

The Background

I've belonged to the most expensive and exclusive health clubs in Los Angeles and Beverly Hills. Year after year I've seen the trainers working with their clients, and year after year I've wondered to myself: Why aren't they losing weight? In fact, why is it that many of them actually get fatter?

Well, the simple truth is that the typical training programs are designed to utilize as much trainer time as possible to generate revenue, but do not incorporate the type of exercises needed to burn calories. Why? Because a trainer can't justify charging for watching you jog on a treadmill or ride a bike, they can only charge you for their personal attention.

This is not to say that trainers have no value. If you need companionship to work on muscle toning, go ahead and keep them. If they are willing to monitor you through your aerobic program at no charge, or you're willing to pay them to do this, go ahead and keep them. But most likely, neither will apply and you'll be going it alone. Great! You need to be listening to upbeat music and burning calories; not wasting your time and hard-earned money.

The Rationale

Most of us lead very busy lives. Finding even one hour per day to exercise is hard enough. The last thing you want is to waste it on an exercise program that burns only 30% of the calories you need to burn in order to lose weight.

Weight loss requires an expenditure of calories in excess of intake. The typical trainer program focuses on muscle building and time churning, not calorie burning through aerobic exercise and conditioning. As will be explained later, what you need is an 80/20 program of aerobics to strengthening. In many cases what the trainers give you is the opposite of what you need!

Basic Facts

Below is a sample of the caloric expenditures for various activities, performed at a moderate pace over a 60-minute period. The examples are for a 150-pound person, and would be more for a heavier person and less for someone lighter. You can get the specifics for your own height and weight at numerous fitness related websites.

- Weight lifting   205 cal/hr

- Yoga   273 cal/hr

- Walking   239 cal/hr

- Bicycling   545 cal/hr

- Stair/stepper/elliptical   409 cal/hr

- Running   682 cal/hr

Most personal training programs involve some form of weight lifting and typically include substantial time wasted on intermittent non-productive gabbing. Some people say they find this form of social interaction motivating, but the end result, unfortunately, is usually far less than 60 minutes of actual exercise. Running, biking, stepping, and other aerobic exercise involve constant activity without rest or social time. The end result: far greater caloric expenditure (two to four times greater) than what would be realized in a typical personal training program.

Celebrity Trainers

So why is it that the stars and other celebrities swear by their Personal Trainers? Let's face it, the type of training a celebrity receives is likely to be far different from what you receive at your local gym.

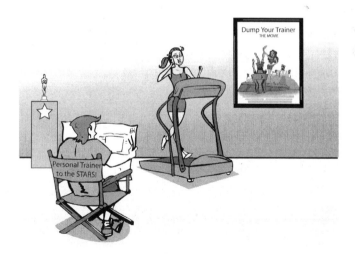

"What do I care if he sits on his ass half the time, the studio's paying."

The typical star trainer is hired to provide a complete exercise program with targeted results. They carefully monitor their clients through all aspects of a regimen. This means they not only work on the strengthening and conditioning phases, but closely monitor clients through their aerobic component as well. So, in essence, celebrity trainers provide a balanced program of aerobic exercise and weight training because their clients (or the production company) are capable of paying for the additional aerobic monitoring. Of course, you could do the same, but at five times the cost – and, realistically, how many of us can afford that? The average trainer charges $50–$100 per hour. So, a complete program of aerobic conditioning and weight training would be prohibitive for the average person.

For example: A supervised exercise program similar to those on the popular TV show *The Biggest Loser* would require 30–50 hours per week, and each week would cost in the neighborhood of $2000–$4000. That's about $1000 per pound! How many pounds were you looking to lose (10, 20, 50)?

The Pitch

Knowing that the average client could never afford this total lifestyle monitoring, personal trainers convince you that somehow you'll find the time to do the aerobic work on your own, and that they will work with you only on the strengthening component.

Of course, in many cases, you won't find the extra time; even worse, you'll go through your day thinking that you've met your caloric goals with just the strength training. You'll think that you can eat at restaurants, have an extra slice of this or that, a few chips, or some other treat, under the false assumption that you've worked with your trainer and can indulge yourself as a reward. But the fact is your caloric expenditure will have been inadequate to offset the calories consumed, and you'll gain more weight – not lose it.

Consider the following scenario: You work with your trainer for an hour. You expend 150–250 calories. You then have a double-scoop ice cream cone (400 calories) to reward yourself. The net result is you've taken in approximately 150 calories more than you've expended. Over time, these added calories will turn into ounces, and then into pounds.

The Weight Loss Formula to Remember

Calories Expended MUST EXCEED Calories Consumed

This formula applies no matter what diet you follow, regardless of carbohydrate (good carb/bad carb), fat, or protein content. Later in the book, we'll discuss our own preferred diet plans to augment your fitness program, but you should always remember that the only way to lose weight naturally is to expend more calories than you consume. There is absolutely no way around this rule, other than surgery.

Studies have indicated that in order to lose weight most expeditiously, a person needs to expend at least 1500–2500 extra calories per week while keeping the calories consumed unchanged. Working with a trainer five times per week will expend a total of 1000 calories and give you a false sense of security. Five sessions of running, biking, stepping, or Cardio Dance will meet this goal, and will improve your cardiovascular health, as well.

Summing up our main ideas

The reasons to dump the trainers:

- They're too expensive and can be a big waste of your time and money

- Their programs often will not help you lose weight.

- The time spent in their programs will prevent you from entering programs that will really work.

- Ultimately, their programs will not improve your cardiovascular health.

That said, there are some situations which may justify a person working with a trainer. These could include:

- You're rich, and can afford to hire them to snooze through your 40-minute aerobic program while waiting for your 20-minute toning segment.

- You're looking to be a hulk and couldn't give a damn about aerobic exercise.

- You have an injury or health condition and are working with a physical therapist as your trainer, under advisement from your doctor.

- You have lots of free time, already have a daily routine of aerobic exercise, and wish to augment this program with one directed by a trainer.

- You need someone cute to count to twelve for you.

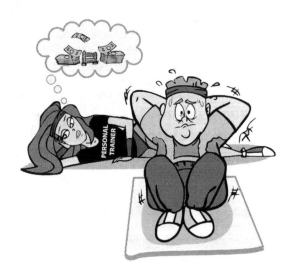

"One, two, three..."

In the first two chapters, we'll explore some of the myths and misinformation of personal training. Later, we'll show you how to be your own Personal Trainer, kick-start your metabolism, and feel great without wasting your money on ineffective personal training.

The Trainer Tells All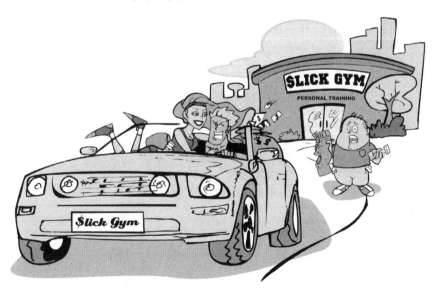

Ten Myths of Personal Training

MYTH #1: You Need a Personal Trainer to Get in Shape

Want to save big bucks and get physically fit? Don't hire me or any other personal trainer. There, I've just come out and said it. You don't need me or any other trainer to achieve your health and fitness goals. Why would I want to share this with you? I am reaching out to you as someone who works as a personal trainer and knows the realities of the industry. I am also someone who has seen more dramatic and sustainable health improvement from other programs that truly work, and won't prey on your insecurities while emptying your wallet.

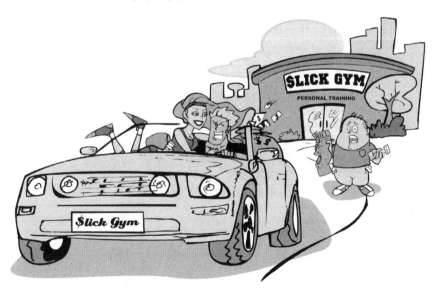

With the current health crisis facing many Americans, wouldn't it make sense if each health seeker had a personal trainer to get them back on track? In this chapter, I will share with you why the answer is a big fat NO!

It's estimated that 65 percent of adult Americans are overweight, and 30 percent of these are obese. Approximately 69 percent of overweight Americans are trying to either lose weight or control their weight. Many are shelling out big bucks to hire PTs (personal trainers). I see these unsuspecting health seekers on a daily basis, and have been hired by many of them. I care about their health and your health. I truly believe in improving one's quality of life through health and fitness. This is why I am telling you to save your money; educate and empower yourself with the understanding that you can be your own personal trainer.

There are many roads to improved health, fitness, and overall well-being. Later in this book, I'll share with you effective, proven and inexpensive strategies to achieve your goals without wasting time and money on personal training sessions.

MYTH #2: Personal Trainers Are Worth the Money

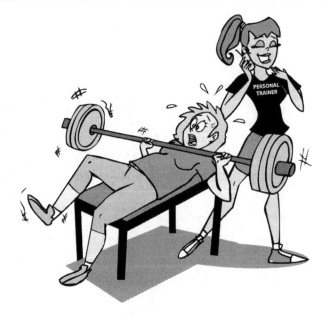

Let's look at a typical one-hour session spent with a trainer. If you frequent gyms, you are no stranger to the following scenario:

Client: "Mary" Age: 42. Weight: 150. Goals: Lose 15 lbs., flatten stomach, tighten thighs.

Trainer: "John" Age: 28. Qualifications: A four-hour online course/CPR. Goal: $$$

The Program

- ✓ **7:03 a.m.: Meet and greet**. John struts up like a runway model, with a genuine look of interest: "Hey, Mary. Sorry I'm late, my dog got sick. You look great! I think we're really making some progress. Let's review your card."

- ✓ **7:10 a.m.: First Exercise:** Three sets of squats with rest in between.

- ✓ **7:15 a.m.: Wait for machine.** John stifles a yawn. Mary: "Yeah, my Peanut is getting old, too..."

- ✓ **7:18 a.m.: Chest Extension:** Three sets with rest in between.

- ✓ **7:25 a.m.: Water Break: Idle chatter**. Mary: "I can give you the number of my vet, she's the best..."

- ✓ **7:29 a.m.:** Mary maneuvers awkwardly into the leg press while John rolls his eyes.

- ✓ **7:30 a.m.: Begin Leg Press:** Three sets with rest in between. Mary is gasping and grimacing at the floor. John, checking out the hot bodies through the aerobics room window: "Just a few more, push it...your legs are getting really strong."

- ✓ **7:35 a.m.: Seated Rows:** Three sets with rest in between. Mary scans her legs. "You know, I really wanted to trim down my thighs..." John, behind her, rolls his eyes.

- ✓ **7:40 a.m.: Biceps Curls with Forward Lunges:** Three sets with rest between sets. Mary, flirting a bit now: "Any plans for the weekend?" John: "I think I need to keep a close eye on Sparky."

- ✓ **7:48 a.m.: Triceps Extension:** Three sets with rest in between. Mary: "I'm not going out of town this weekend. Gas is just too expensive... Are you going to be around?"

- ✓ **7:50 a.m.: Abdominals:** Three minutes of medicine ball crunches. John: "I'm gonna be spending all weekend with my 'drama partner,' Nicole. We've both got auditions and have to rehearse our love scene for *Passions*.

- ✓ **7:53 a.m.: Stretch.** John: "Great work today, you're really getting strong. I think we should extend your program."

- ✓ **7:59 a.m.: Running her credit card.** Mary: "Good luck with your audition. See you on Monday."

Breakdown: 130 Calories Burned; $60 session.

Mary! You could have walked for an hour while listening to upbeat, invigorating music. Calories Burned: 400. Cost: Free! Or even better, taken a free Cardio Dance class at the gym, met new friends and gone through the day feeling sensational. Calories Burned: 650+.

MYTH #3: Personal Trainers Have Certifications from Reputable Organizations

I know from my work that there are many highly skilled, educated, and dedicated Personal Trainers well worth the expense and very appropriate and worthwhile for specific circumstances. This book is not about those elite trainers who work with athletes pursuing excellence or competitive body builders, or those who specializing in physical rehabilitation. Personal training in that arena is completely different. Unfortunately, the vast majority of Personal Trainers found in gyms today are working with a one-size-fits-all mentality and do little more than count repetitions while calculating how to book you for as many sessions as possible.

What is a Certified Personal Trainer?
There are a tremendous number of personal training and fitness certifications available. The standards vary greatly. Some require no more than completing an online course, others offer one-day workshop certifications, and many gyms have their own certifications.

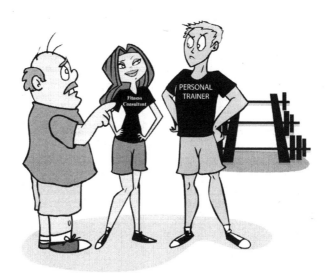

"Weren't you my waiter at El Grande Burrito last night?"

The certifications that are the most reputable are:

- The American College of Sports Medicine (ACSM)

- The American Council (ACE)

- The National Strength and Conditioning Association (NSCA)

- The National Academy of Sports Medicine (NASM)

- Aerobics and Fitness Association of America (AFAA)

Certification from these agencies ensures that your trainer has demonstrated at least a minimum level of knowledge related to proper exercise choice and technique. All of these certifications also require a current certification in CPR.

Tricky Titles

What do all the titles mean? Is there any significance to the way "fitness" professionals identify themselves? For example: "Fitness Consultant" – this title certainly sounds credible. I know a trainer who calls himself a fitness consultant – he's an out-of-work actor with a great body. When I asked him what certifications or education he had, he smiled and said, "Look at my body, I obviously know what I'm doing." So, what do these titles really mean?

Fitness Consultant/Fitness Coordinator

The definition of a consultant is one who provides advice and services presumably as an expert or specialist. In the mega-chain gyms, these commissioned salespeople are sometimes called "Fitness Coordinators." Typically, they're attractive, aggressive, and superficially friendly. They'll ask you a series of basic questions in order to establish a rapport while trying to determine how large a package of personal training they can sell you, along with which type of trainer would "best suit your needs."

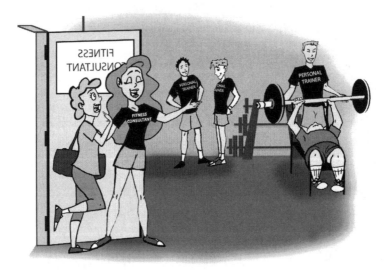

"I don't care about his credentials, just as long as he's tall."

In the smaller, independent gyms, the Fitness Consultants usually function both as a sales rep and the actual Personal Trainer. Anyone can legally call themselves a consultant for almost anything, regardless of their qualifications. There are a few exceptions to this rule, but generally speaking, in the fitness industry, anyone can say they are a Fitness Consultant.

Fitness Professional

A professional is the term used for anyone who possesses advanced knowledge of a profession or trade. Technically, those who are in the fitness industry don't necessarily need to have a nationally recognized fitness certification or a degree based solely on this definition. They're simply expected to look good, know more than the average person about working out, and have a good rapport with the clients.

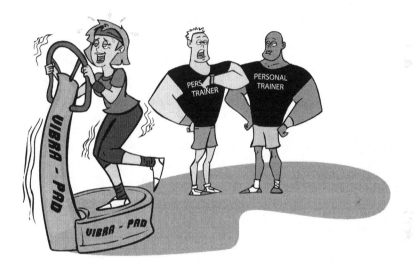

"Five more minutes and I'll be done with her hour of 'personal training'."

In fact, no state has a law in place that requires a personal training certification or a degree in order to be considered a so called fitness professional. Similarly, there are absolutely no governing bodies that oversee the practices of the fitness industry as a whole. There are many individuals and certifying organizations working toward implementing national standards, including State Board Examinations. Perhaps the public will be better protected in the future. Until that happens, the individual consumers of fitness services need to take it upon themselves to be informed and wary of fancy fitness titles.

Fitness Expert

The actual definition of the word expert is "having, involving, or displaying special skill or knowledge derived from training." Again, there is no industry standard, so anyone can make a business card and *voila*! They're a "Fitness Expert."

Some Personal Trainers use elaborate titles so that you'll believe they're worth the money you're paying them. They dread the day you realize you could be exercising more efficiently without them. In the example earlier, Mary could be paying down her mortgage rather than paying John's rent!

A Trainer to "best suit your needs"

In order to ensure your continued patronage, trainers have to develop dependency. This dependency is established by creating relationships based on the following trainer types: friends, intimidators, gurus, and supporters.

The Friends

The "friends" are the popular types we all look up to. These trainers usually have great rapport with their clients and are the entertainers. This is one of the biggest pitfalls of hiring a PT. Paying someone to watch you workout is bad enough, but paying someone to make you laugh while you pretend to workout is denial!

The Intimidator or Drill Sergeant

Another PT strategy is the "intimidator" or "drill sergeant." This trainer keeps clients by intimidation, usually pushing them far past their limits under some variation of the misguided premise of "no pain – no gain."

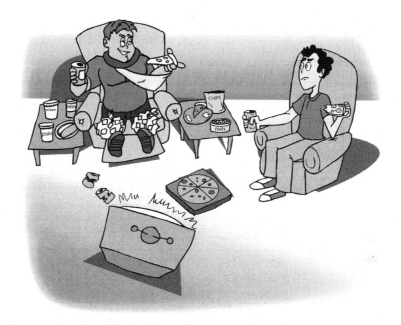

*"Yeah, well, I'm serious about getting back in shape. I train with Big Jack.
Just one session with him and I can't even walk for three days."*

Although you may think the soreness after these sessions is normal, this type of intensity can be counterproductive and may even be dangerous.

The Guru
Every gym has a "guru" trainer who says that his or her style of training is the ONLY way to get results. The guru trainer usually has dedicated disciples accompanied by a huge ego. With so many people looking up to them, they begin to believe they have the perfect fitness formula. If you train with a guru, be prepared to listen. These trainers like to talk: "Every morning I drink six cups of beet juice, before my twelve egg whites..."

The Supporters or Enablers
Finally, we have the "supporters" or "enablers" (many times, these trainers are out of shape themselves). This is the non-intimidating trainer who indulges every excuse: "It is hot today. Let's just do a few stretches." Or "I'm sorry you had such a bad day at work. Let's just put you on the VibraPad."

Two things these trainer types have in common when it comes to getting you in shape: they're not the best use of your time, and the time they spend with you is still going to be expensive.

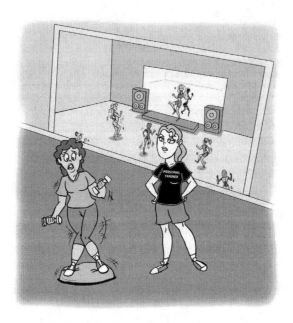

"How many calories does this burn?"

What's a better way to spend your time and energy in pursuit of your goals? Read on, the trainer will tell you more.

MYTH #4: Personal Trainers Know About Nutrition and Supplements

What Should I Eat?

Personal Trainers are asked this question every day, and their enthusiastic clients reflexively accept whatever nutritional advice they receive. Sometimes it's sound advice in line with FDA guidelines, but often the trainers have their own bias toward a particular fad diet which may be unsuitable for a particular client's needs. For example, if a client is a diabetic or has special nutritional needs, these needs should be determined by their personal physician and their diet regulated only by a licensed health care professional.

I've studied nutrition and diet for years, and have hands-on experience designing specific meal plans for hundreds of clients. In my experience, most diets – even fad diets – work, but only for a short time. For long-term success, what a person needs is a realistic lifestyle change that he/she can live with, even when Life Happens.

Life Happens

"Life Happens" could mean anything and everything; from a few too many Friday night margaritas to a three-week, all-you-can (and will)-eat cruise. I often see even my most highly disciplined clients return to me after falling off some ultra-restrictive diet program. They're disillusioned and discouraged after packing on the pounds they worked so hard to lose. They again commit to the latest fad diet plan, feverish with resolve and dedication, swearing each time: "This time I'll stick to it for sure."

Life will always happen. What people need is a realistic approach to eating suited to their lifestyle – not just for two weeks or twelve weeks, but for a lifetime. Can this be done without a trainer? Absolutely! Later on, I'll show you how to combine a sane and solid exercise program with my delicious, balanced, and nutritious "Real-life Meal Plan" that you can follow and manage on your own.

Supplements

Be wary of trainers pushing certain diet products. Diet and nutrition supplements are HUGE moneymakers for many corporate gyms. Trainers are often pressured or given incentives to sell supplements – supplements that have no proven benefits, and some of which can even be harmful.

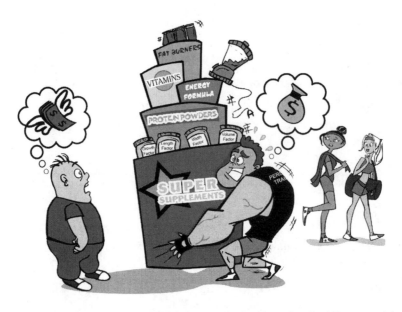

"All natural" diet pills, herbal supplements, and "fat-burning" pills are a big business in this country, with little or no evidence of their effectiveness. Also, many contain amphetamine-like stimulants which can result in serious health complications, including heart attacks, seizures, and death.

In May 2004, *Consumer Reports* reported on twelve supplements found commonly in health stores, which it labeled the "dirty dozen." Complications of taking these supplements included cancer, kidney failure, heart and respiratory problems, and liver failure. The reader is referred to the article, which is listed in the References.

MYTH #5 & MYTH #6: Personal Trainers Care About Your Progress; Personal Trainers Want You to Be Self-Sufficient

Tracking Your Progress
One of the primary reasons people hire Personal Trainers is to track their progress.

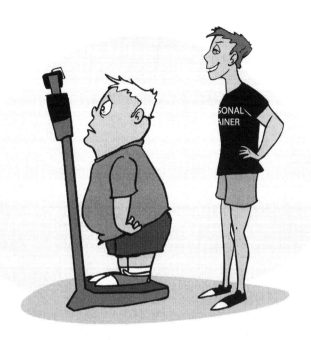

"See, you've already lost five pounds of fat and gained ten pounds of muscle."

In order to map that progress, trainers need to quantifiably track you, evaluating weight, body measurements, body fat testing, strength, heart rate recovery, and many other time-consuming, yet important tests to record your level.

I have a few clients that prefer to be kept accountable with weekly weight measurements, but surprisingly, many of my clients are not interested in being pinched, weighed, and measured every two weeks. Without these regular measurements, though, there is really no way I can accurately record their progress. Many trainers don't offer more than a weigh-in and, occasionally, an (often inaccurate) body fat percentage calculation. Many offer nothing at all.

Isn't it important to make sure your program is achieving the results you want? For many trainers, the answer is a surprising NO! Why? Because reaching your goal weight will only make your trainer more "dumpable." Of course, conversely, if you're not making progress toward your goal that is exactly why you should dump your trainer in the first place.

Trainers know this, so many hide behind these familiar phrases: Sometimes the scale goes up when you are putting on so much muscle; but you look a lot leaner; next week, let's try lighter weights so you won't get bulky muscles; it's not important to look at the scale, just think about how tight you feel.

You should be losing weight, if that's your goal. You should have a trainer who records your weekly progress and provides evidence that the program is really working – not one who just provides lip service by saying that you look great. Better yet, dump your trainer and do it on your own.

Myth #7: Personal Trainers Design Time-Efficient, Effective Workouts

The Client's Logic
Your goal: Lose 30 lbs.

You're busy. You want the most time-efficient and effective exercise program, so you hire a personal trainer to get you in shape quickly. You are ready to get in the best shape of your life, fast. You pick a headshot from the "Trainer Wall of Fame" and schedule your session.

Trainer's Logic
Trainer's goal: Sell training sessions. How many sessions per week will client X book with me? One thing is for sure, when client X reaches their goal, I'm out of a job. Better start off 'befriending' him. It'll take at least six months before he sees results: Cha-ching!

Time-Efficient Training Sessions
The first session left you sweat-less. Your new trainer talked a lot about your specifically designed program, your body type, your training goals, and your lack of "core stability." You thought you were ready to work out. Oh, no – the trainer explains that you need to slowly go through each level of the training model. This will take months.

The trainer asks you to sign a contract and prepay for eight sessions, asking "Aren't you committed to this?" Your head is spinning, you feel discouraged about your current fitness level, and maybe this is what you have to do to get in shape. You prepay for the sessions. Gotcha!

Progress

Now that you've purchased the sessions, you realize it isn't easy to coordinate your busy schedule with the trainer's – merely making the appointment feels like a workout. You finally meet at the gym to train, and spend the first 15 minutes talking about your progress and doing "balance" exercises, followed by rolling around on a piece of foam that looks like a pool toy. You leave the session without breaking a sweat, and as you drive home, you try to rationalize the time you spent at the gym: "Well, the trainer said I need to build my endurance slowly before I can move on to the second block."

Thirty days later, $480 spent on your first eight sessions and…NOTHING! You haven't lost any weight, you haven't lost any inches, but you have lost time and money, and now you're discouraged. So what do you do? You eat!

Time-Efficient, Effective Program to Lose 30 Pounds

If you want to lose weight, your trainer should have recommended a cardio-intensive program: 40–60 minutes of aerobic exercise followed by 10–15 minutes of strength training and five minutes of stretching. With this program, you would have lost eight to ten pounds in the first 30 days, and you could have done it for free. The problem is the trainer isn't necessary for that training protocol; they have to waste your time in order to make money.

Don't blame the trainer for trying to make a living, but you can blame him/her for conning you into a program that doesn't work. A truly legitimate trainer would have recognized that your time is limited and would have designed a program to maximize your aerobic workout, even if it meant minimizing his/her role in the short run (i.e., 40 minutes of aerobics followed by 15–20 minutes of toning – not an hour). Ultimately, through your positive results, he/she would have developed a relationship with you that lasts.

MYTH #8 & MYTH #9: Personal Trainers Practice What They Preach; Personal Trainers Are Healthy Role Models

Personal Trainers may not be training themselves the way they train you. Most trainers I know do far more cardio training and far less weight training than their clients. They practice a routine similar to the 80/20 rule which is more time-efficient and burns more calories – making their muscles stand out and creating a lean enough body mass to actually bring out an otherwise fat-concealed six-pack.

Steroids

There are many dangerous trends in bodybuilding and fitness modeling. Unfortunately, many trainers promote a "healthy lifestyle" while making themselves sick in order to compete and model. Despite the serious health consequences (impotence, high blood pressure, heart palpitations, and jaundice – to name just a few), many people seeking a naturally unattainable physique turn to steroids. The lure of steroids and other growth-enhancing drugs has drawn in many who yearn to have the sculpted bodies featured in magazines.

Diuretics

Bodybuilders dehydrate themselves with diuretics in order to make muscles bulge as much as possible; some competitive bodybuilders even have a glass of wine right before going onstage. Dehydration puts severe strain on your internal organs and affects your mental capacity.

Fat Burners

Another dirty secret among those seeking naturally unattainable bodies is the use of "fat burners." Even after the ban on Ephedra, a component of many fat burners is Ma Huang, the plant from which ephedrine is derived and which can be just as dangerous. Many runners, bodybuilders, and other athletes take these supplements to enhance their performance, without realizing or accepting the potentially hazardous effects.

Over-Training

Many serious athletes become so obsessed with working out that they end up training too often and not resting between workouts. This "over-training" can lead to general fatigue, irritability, moodiness, depression, anxiety, decreased appetite, and possibly impaired immune function. Getting too much exercise can be as bad as getting too little. It can lead to injuries, degenerative and arthritic changes, as well as other long-term health, psychological, and emotional problems.

MYTH #10: Personal Trainers Are Qualified To Handle Medical and Psychological Problems

In addition to not getting real and sustainable advice on diets, many clients mistake their trainers for doctors and go to them for medical advice. Consider the following: "My knee really hurts; should I work out today?" Don't ask a Personal Trainer, because he/she will probably make something up instead of referring you to a medical professional. As mentioned earlier, a trainer needs to be useful to you in order to get paid. Why would he/she tell you: "I don't know, ask a doctor"? Personal Trainers should never give medical advice, but I often hear trainers explaining the intricacies of the intervertebral discs and giving advice on what to do after back surgery.

Personal trainers (usually) are not MD's or therapists, but their clients often feel comfortable sharing personal information. Personal Training is very intimate and the client can be vulnerable. We don't usually let strangers touch our bodies, tell them what we hate most about ourselves, or confide that we ate a pint of Ben and Jerry's recently after we broke up, issues for which they have no training.

Some clients have serious eating disorders, depression, or other psychological problems. Even well-meaning personal trainers can inadvertently give advice instead of referring their clients to medical professionals.

Be Your Own Personal Trainer

Throughout this book, I'll provide you with the resources you need to be your own Personal Trainer. I'll show you why dumping your trainer and investing in yourself is the best option for your bottom line, as well as for your waistline.

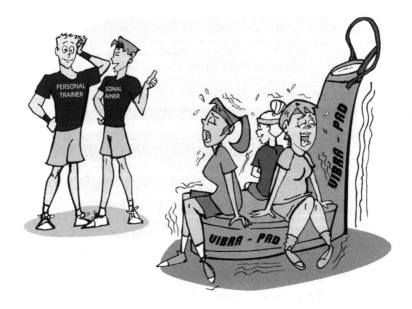

"The gym owner calls it 'group personal training'."

Celebrity Diets

The pressure for celebrities to have perfect bodies often leads to unhealthy and extreme dieting. It's unfortunate that many stick-thin actresses claim to eat healthy diets and exercise with their trainers regularly. I find that impossible to believe. Subsisting on a diet of caffeine, nicotine, and an occasional calorie does not provide enough energy for basic bodily functions, let alone exercise.

Many women I've trained get discouraged that they can't attain the size 0 that they see on TV or in magazines. They often feel "fat," although they are at an ideal weight, with body composition, are exercising regularly, and are eating a nutritious diet. It is important to understand that just because someone looks incredibly thin; it doesn't mean they are lean or healthy. Extreme dieters often lose lean muscle, altering their body composition and increasing their body fat percentage. Even though they are a low body weight, they are Skinny Fat. It is important to question images in the media and to remember health, energy, and happiness are not found in thinness.

Many celebrities suffer from eating disorders or have adopted disordered eating behaviors to maintain such low body weights.

Here's a look at the dangerous, difficult, diligent, and disorders of celebrity weight loss.

The Dangerous

Master Cleanse
The "Master Cleanse" is a fast that requires subsisting for 10 or more days solely on fresh-squeezed lemon juice, cayenne pepper, maple syrup, and water.

Beyoncé Knowles
Announced that she had lost 20 pounds on the fast to prepare for her starring role in the film *Dreamgirls*.

"I lived on water, cayenne pepper, and maple syrup for 14 days. It was tough; everyone was eating and I was dying." – Beyoncé Knowles on *Oprah*, 2006

The One Meal Per Day Plan

Liz Hurley

Reportedly lost post baby weight with the Caveman Diet. This diet relies on the theory that we don't need three meals a day. She ate just one meal a day and never mixed proteins with carbohydrates.

Victoria Beckham

Reportedly eats one meal a day, consisting of steamed fish, vegetables, and salad, in order to maintain her painfully thin figure.

Mariah Carey

Purple Food Diet

Reportedly, three days a week she eats nothing but grapes, plums, beetroots, and other purple-hued foods.

Sarah Michelle Gellar

Cabbage Soup Diet

Reportedly ate cabbage soup for seven days, along with fruit, vegetables, fish, and chicken. Sarah Michelle claimed to lose 30 lbs.

The Smoking Weight Loss Plan?

We all know better – smoking kills. Unfortunately, smoking is also viewed as an appetite suppressant, and many desperate to lose weight will do anything – including risk their health – to do so.

Who "Lights Up to Lighten Up"

- Jennifer Aniston
- Drew Barrymore
- Neve Campbell
- Sheryl Crow
- Claire Danes
- Johnny Depp
- Cameron Diaz
- Shannon Daugherty

- Minnie Driver
- Colin Farrell
- Lindsay Lohan
- Courtney Love
- Kate Moss
- Sarah Jessica Parker
- Michelle Pfiefer
- Joaquin Phoenix
- Christina Ricci

The Difficult

THE RAW FOOD DIET
Followers of the Raw Food Diet eat only uncooked food.

- Alicia Silverstone
- Carol Alt
- Demi Moore
- Woody Harrelson
- Sting
- Seal
- Uma Thurman

THE MACROBIOTIC DIET
The Macrobiotic Diet includes whole grains such as rice and quinoa, fresh vegetables and fruits, seaweeds, and fermented foods such as soy. Followers avoid processed foods.

- Madonna
- Courtney Love
- Gwyneth Paltrow

The Diligent Zone Followers
Barry Sears invented the Zone Diet. It advises eating a specific ratio of carbohydrates, protein, and fats: specifically 40 percent: 30 percent: 30 percent.

Ideally, every meal and snack should provide 40 percent of calories from carbohydrate, 30 percent from protein, and 30 percent from fat. This is what some Zone fans call the 40:30:30 plan.

- Jennifer Aniston
- Sandra Bullock
- Cindy Crawford
- Sarah Jessica Parker
- Brad Pitt
- Rene Zelleweger

Why Can't I Look Like That?
You Can…Get Photoshop

It's an illusion – the flawlessness skin, perfect hair, flat stomachs, fuller breasts, pumped lips, and toned muscles. These robotic magazine images often perpetuate unrealistic ideals. Although we know that magazine covers and photos are retouched, the images still leave many feeling hopeless and defeated. I've had clients bring me images of celebrity body parts they cut out of magazines, hoping to achieve the jiggle-free arms or flat stomach. The focus on perfection is counterproductive; remember, an entire team of hair, makeup, lighting, and retouching professionals were required to create that photograph.

Happily, there is a backlash to all of this retouching. Some celebrities like Kate Winslet don't want their images drastically altered. Advertising campaigns, like DOVE, are emphasizing "real women," and there are now a new generation of fitness magazines, which are using true life "reader models," and thus creating healthier, more realistic role models.

Eating Disorders

Many celebrities suffer from eating disorders or have adopted disordered eating behaviors to maintain such low body weights.

Anorexia and Bulimia
Anorexia nervosa is a complex psychological eating disorder. There are new rumors every week about which celebrities are anorexic. Is she or isn't she…? Being skinny

does not necessarily imply that one has anorexia. Anorexia is an eating disorder where people literally starve themselves. It usually begins in young people around the onset of puberty. People suffering from anorexia are very skinny, but are convinced that they are overweight. Since they believe they are overweight, they refuse to eat, often developing serious medical complications that sometimes result in death.

Bulimia nervosa is a psychological condition in which a person engages in binge eating followed by intentional purging. Purging can take the form of vomiting, the use of laxatives, diuretics or other medication, or excessive exercise. Today eating disorders constitute a major health concern. According to the National Eating Disorders Organization, between 5 million and 10 million girls and women, and 2 million boys and men have some type of eating disorder. As many as 15 percent of the men and women, boys and girls, who are diagnosed as having anorexia nervosa will die from that disorder. An amazing 1 out of 5 college-aged women are engaging in some form of bulimic behavior (binging and purging).

If you think you may suffer from anorexia or bulimia, please get the help you need.

http://www.nationaleatingdisorders.org

Some well-known actress have confirmed their struggles with anorexia and bulimia, others vehemently deny the accusations that they have an eating disorder.

Jamie-Lynn DiScala, actress
Battled severe anorexia and "exercise bulimia" in high school, wrote a book about it (2002's *Wise Girl*), and is now a spokeswoman for the National Eating Disorders Association.

"I was fortunate enough in that I could afford therapists, psychiatrists and nutritionists." *New York Post*

Calista Flockhart, actress
The former *Ally McBeal* star told *People* in 1988:

"I'm not too thin. Am I anorexic? I guess my answer would have to be no."

Later she admitted that she struggled with anorexia while filming the show.

"I started under-eating, over-exercising, pushing myself too hard and brutalizing my immune system."

Courtney Thorne-Smith, actress
Battled an eating disorder and developed anorexia due to the pressure to be thin. Her slide into anorexia led her to quit the television show *Ally Mc Beal*.

"The amount of time I spent thinking about food and being upset about my body was insane." *People*

Portia de Rossi, actress
Admitted to *Vogue* magazine that she struggled with anorexia while starring on the hit show *Ally McBeal*.

"I've often wondered if I wasn't on that show if [anorexia] may not have happened. I didn't really know at that point what it was like to be a celebrity, and the only people I knew at the time who had a similar experience were these women whom I worked with. They became my role models."

Tracey Gold, actress
Sought treatment for anorexia. "All life meant was losing weight, counting calories." *People*, 1994

Christina Ricci, actress
"I did get all my tips from a Tracey Gold Lifetime movie on anorexia. It taught me what to do." *Jane*, 2002

Billy Bob Thornton, actor
"Frankly, for a while there, I think I had a little mental problem," said Thornton, who lost 59 pounds. "I got anorexic; of course I denied it to my girlfriend and everyone else who said I had an eating disorder." *LA Daily News*, 1998

Victoria Beckham (Posh Spice), singer
"I was very obsessed. I mean, I could tell you the fat content and the calorie content in absolutely anything. I was never anorexic, I was never bulimic, but I was probably very close to it." ABC's *20/20*, 2003

Ashlee Simpson, singer

"I was around a lot of girls with eating disorders, and I actually had a minor one myself. It was about six months of not eating too much at all." *Cosmopolitan*, 2005

Mary-Kate Olsen

Mary-Kate Olsen has sought treatment for anorexia.

Nicole Richie

Nicole Richie repeatedly denies that she suffers from an eating disorder.

Don't look to celebrities as health and fitness role models. Instead, set realistic health goals and focus on your personal fitness needs.

The Dump Your Trainer Diet & Fitness Program

The Simple and Fun Way to Rapid Weight Loss and Long-term Fitness

The Basics

First

Get cleared by your doctor. The worst thing you can do is hurt yourself, so before you start any exercise program make sure you get a complete checkup from your doctor, including an evaluation of your spine, knees, and hips. I would also advise a diagnostic evaluation by a cardiologist, particularly if you are over 40 or if there is any history of cardiovascular disease in your family.

Second

Understand your limitations and start off slowly. The worst thing you can do is injure yourself – SO DON'T DO IT. The last thing you need is to be laid up with an injury, depressed, and eating chips and guacamole.

Please don't risk permanent damage to your joints, spine, ligaments and heart using injury prone, media hyped 'fitness' programs designed to generate TV ratings, not long-term health.

It's normal to have a slight amount of tightness in your muscles when starting an exercise program. If you're tight with pain the day after, then you overdid it, and you need to cut back at least 50% on the intensity (not duration) of your program.

Pep Talk Time! Let's Make a Plan!

In order to reach your health and fitness goals, you must have a road map to follow.

Step One

Start by asking yourself how much total weight do you want to lose? You can use the following charts as a general guide to a healthy weight.

Height and Weight Table for Women

Frame Size

Height	Small	Medium	Large
4' 10"	102-111	109-121	118-131
4' 11"	103-113	111-123	120-134
5' 0"	104-115	113-126	122-137
5' 1"	106-118	115-129	125-140
5' 2"	108-121	118-132	128-143
5' 3"	111-124	121-135	131-147
5' 4"	114-127	124-138	134-151
5' 5"	117-130	127-141	137-155
5' 6"	120-133	130-144	140-159
5' 7"	123-136	133-147	143-163
5' 8"	126-139	136-150	146-167
5' 9"	129-142	139-153	149-170
5' 10"	132-145	142-156	152-173
5' 11"	135-148	145-159	155-176
6' 0"	138-151	148-162	158-179

Height and Weight Table for Men

Frame Size

Height	Small	Medium	Large
5' 2"	128-134	131-141	138-150
5' 3"	130-136	133-143	140-153
5'' 4"	132-138	135-145	142-156
5' 5"	134-140	137-148	144-160
5' 6"	136-142	139-151	146-164
5' 7"	138-145	142-154	149-168
5' 8"	140-148	145-157	152-172
5' 9"	142-151	148-160	155-176
5' 10"	144-154	151-163	158-180
5' 11"	146-157	154-166	161-184
6' 0"	149-160	157-170	164-188
6' 1"	152-164	160-174	168-192
6' 2"	155-168	164-178	172-197
6' 3"	158-172	167-182	176-202
6' 4"	162-176	171-187	181-207

*Ideal Weights per the Metropolitan Life Insurance Company (1983).

What size is your frame?

If you are left-handed, extend your right arm. If you are right-handed, extend your left arm. With your free hand, wrap your thumb and middle finger (yes, the one that some people use when in heavy traffic) around your extended wrist. Be sure to wrap it around the SMALLEST section of your wrist – very close to the base of your hand.

Small Frame: If your middle finger and thumb overlap, you have a small frame.

Medium Frame: If your middle finger and thumb touch, you have a medium frame.

Large Frame: If your middle finger and thumb do not meet, you have a large frame.

Your next step is to set a reasonable weight loss pace for yourself. You can base your own pace on any number of factors, including the results of the fitness assessment we offer later on in this chapter, but a great place to start would be the general recommendations from the American College of Sports Medicine, which are one to two pounds per week.

<u>Step Two - Eating Plan</u>

First, look at your eating habits, such as when you eat, what you eat, how much you eat, where you eat, and how often you eat. If you feel out of control, start by keeping a journal and write down everything you eat. Seeing it on paper helps put the numbers in perspective and will help you gain control.

Plan all of your meals. Yes, it's a lot of work at first, but the extra effort really creates the discipline you need to stick with it long-term. Get on track by shopping only with a list. Get yourself on an eating schedule that has you eating small, balanced meals or snacks every two to three hours.

Finding the Best Diet for YOU

The message of this book is that YOU can be your best fitness trainer. You know your body better than anyone. You should care about your body and health more than anyone. It has been said our bodies are our curriculum for life. We can listen to and learn from our bodies to achieve invigorating health to enjoy all areas of our lives.

It is similar to the notion that you must be your own best money manager. You may be able to find professionals to help you in this area, consultants and interested family members too, but at the end of the day, you need to know the numbers to make sure your interests are being looked after.

The more you know about your own body, the way it works, what makes it feel good, how it is a unique gift, the more empowered you will be in all areas of your life. This means you have to be keenly aware of what you put in your body and how nutrition is a key component to your health.

When I work with clients and have them keep daily food logs, not only to keep track of calories, but also to increase their awareness of how certain foods affect how they feel. It is exciting to realize that a simple food allergy may be the cause of your extra stomach bloating or a daily headache can be eliminating by avoiding certain foods or additives. I have learned from my clients and seen firsthand how powerful simple changes can greatly improve well-being and weight loss.

We need to be conscious of how food affects us, the best way to figure out if you are having negative reactions to foods is to experiment and keep a log of how you feel if you eliminate certain foods and additives. For example, I was working with a woman who was motivated to lose weight for her wedding. She was experiencing terrible headaches every day, stress seemed to be a logical conclusion, but after looking at her food logs, I noticed that she was consuming over ten packets of artificial sweetener per day. She had never used artificial sweetener prior to her wedding weight loss program. I have always been an advocate of a clean, chemical free diet full of organic fruits and vegetables, so I recommend she eliminate the artificial sweeteners and in less than a week she was free of her headaches.

Your body is always talking to you so listen and observe how you feel after eating.

You control what you put in your body and therefore you should take the time of knowing what you are ingesting. Many trainers will not go over this with you and some trainers even endorse diets products that are full of chemicals simply because they are low in calories. I will share information with you here that I have learned, but it is my hope that you learn more on your own and continue listening to your body.

What type of diet will give you the greatest amount of energy, health and help you maintain your ideal weight? The answer is different for each of us.

Each one of us needs to experiment to find the "right" diet. I've trained people who feel best on high protein diets others who swear by raw food diets and many who maintain their ideal weight by watching their portions while enjoying a variety of foods.

If you are open to trying new ways of eating, go for it! Try out a vegetarian (someone who eats no animals (no cows, pigs, chickens, fish, etc.), vegan (eats no animal products (no animals, dairy, eggs, etc.) or a raw food list (who eats only raw foods?).

If you choose to experiment with a new way of eating pay close attention to how you feel, you may be surprised at an increase in your energy as you eliminate processed foods.

Follow these basic guidelines with any type of diet plan you choose:

✓ Eat a wide variety of whole foods. Foods that are in their natural form with the least possible processing.

✓ Eat sufficient, high quality low-fat proteins.

✓ Try to consume 1-cup fresh fruit and 4-6 cups fresh vegetables daily.

✓ Be moderate with your starch intake (carbohydrates) bread, rice, corn breads and pastas).

✓ Reduce animal fats and eliminate hydrogenated and processed oils. Eliminate processed snack foods (chips, cookies, crackers, cakes…)

Possible Food Allergies

Artificial Colors
Artificial Sweeteners
Beer
Chocolate
Coffee
Cane Sugar
Dairy Products
Eggs
Gluten (a protein found in wheat, rye, barley, and oats)
Legumes

MSG (Monosodium glutamate, a common food additive)

Nightshades (tomatoes, potatoes, eggplant, peppers, tobacco)

Nuts (all kinds)

Seeds

Strawberries

Wheat

Yeast

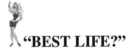

"BEST LIFE?"

Bob Greene, Oprah's Personal Trainer and Author, endorses chemically sweetened foods on his "Best Life" food list. Many of the foods on his list contain artificial ingredients. If you're trying to avoid artificial ingredients and colors then you may want to avoid some of the "Best Life" products. I don't think it's the "Best Life" Choice.

Compare the ingredients of my favorite yogurt, FAGE Non-Fat Greek Yogurt vs. Bob Greene's "Best Life" Yoplait Light:

Yoplait Light

INGREDIENTS: Milk Non-Fat Grade A Pasteurized Cultured, Fructose, Corn Starch Modified, Strawberries, Blueberries, Raspberries, Whey Protein Concentrate, Gelatin Kosher, Whey, Citric Acid, Tri Calcium Phosphate, Aspartame, Potassium Sorbate To Retain Freshness, Natural Flavor(s), Red 40, Blue 1

Nutrition Facts:
Serving Size 1 container
Servings Per Container about 1
Amount Per Serving
Calories 100
Total Fat 0g
Cholesterol 5mg
Sodium 85mg
Total Carbohydrate 17g
Dietary Fiber 0g
Sugars 11g
Protein 5g

Or:

FAGE, Non Fat Greek Yogurt

INGREDIENTS: Nonfat strained yogurt made from Grade A pasteurized skimmed milk, live active yogurt cultures (L.Bulgaricus, S.Thermophilus

Nutrition Facts:
Servings Per Container about 1
Amount Per Serving
Calories 80
Total Fat 0 g
Cholesterol 0mg
Sodium 55mg
Total Carbohydrate 6g
Dietary Fiber 0
Sugars 6g
Protein 13g

Step Three - Exercise Plan

Start out slow; you don't want to burn yourself out after the first week. If you aren't currently working out, aim for two or three sessions per week. Once you feel comfortable with three sessions, keep adding every two weeks until you're exercising five days a week.

Keep in mind that the four important components of your workout program are:

- Frequency
- Duration
- Intensity
- Type (Mode)

Frequency of Exercise
The first component of cardiovascular exercise is frequency of the exercise, which refers to the number of exercise sessions per week. To improve both cardiovascular fitness and to decrease body fat or maintain body fat at optimum levels, you should do cardiovascular exercise at least three days a week. The American College of Sports Medicine recommends three to five days a week for most cardiovascular programs. Those of you who are very out of shape and/or who are overweight and doing weight-bearing cardiovascular exercise, such as an aerobics class or jogging,

might want to have at least 36–48 hours of rest between workouts, in order to prevent an injury and to promote adequate bone and joint stress recovery.

Duration of Exercise

The second component of cardiovascular exercise is the duration, which refers to the time you've spent exercising. The cardiovascular session, not including the warm up and cool down, should vary from 20–60 minutes to gain significant cardio-respiratory and fat-burning benefits.

It is important that you gradually increase the duration before you increase the intensity. For example, when beginning a walking program, be more concerned with increasing the number of minutes of the exercise session before you increase the intensity by increasing your speed or by walking hilly terrain.

Types of Exercise (Mode)

Aerobic Exercise – Cardiovascular Strength Training – Muscular Strength and Endurance Exercise – Flexibility – Stretching and Warm-up Exercises

Intensity (How Hard You Are Working Out)

One of the most common mistakes new exercisers make is in not measuring exercise intensity. You might make the mistake of working too hard (which can lead to injury and burnout), or not working hard enough (which can lead to frustration from lack of results).

There are different ways to measure your intensity. The most common ways are:

Target Heart Rate

Rate of Perceived Exertion (RPE) – how easily can you speak while you're exercising? *See section "alternative to target heart rates."*

Fitness Assessment

Usually, during a first or second personal training session you should have been given a fitness assessment to determine your current fitness level. Although many clients opt not to do the fitness assessment, I recommend it as a good way to establish your baseline and help track your progress. But you can do all the basic assessments on your own – so grab a stopwatch and get ready.

Before starting or continuing any exercise program, ask yourself some basic questions:

1. What is my current level of fitness and physical activity?

2. What are my fitness goals?

3. What is my daily resting heart rate?

4. What is my maximum heart rate?

For a beginning exerciser, a sensible goal is to improve overall health and to adapt to a more active, energetic lifestyle. Beginners should monitor their heart rate and train aerobically (80% of maximum or below) for at least the first three months of their program. Heart rate zones may be determined by using the 220 or 226 minus age formula. More experienced exercisers may have goals like performance improvement or body composition changes. These entail designing an annual calendar of workout according to heart rate guidelines, and regular performance testing to monitor overtraining and improvement.

According to the American Medical Association, your maximum heart rate is approximately 220 minus your age. Your target heart rate is generally between 50 and 75 percent of your maximum heart rate. This is your ideal heart rate to reach during aerobic exercise such as brisk walking or jogging.

Target Heart Rates

AHA Recommendation
Health professionals know the importance of proper pacing during exercise. To receive the benefits of physical activity, it's important not to tire too quickly. Pacing yourself is especially important if you've been inactive.

Target heart rates let you measure your initial fitness level and monitor your progress in a fitness program. This approach requires measuring your pulse periodically as you exercise and staying within 50–85 percent of your maximum heart rate. This range is called your target heart rate.

What is an alternative to target heart rates?

Some people can't measure their pulse or don't want to take their pulse when exercising. If this is true for you, try using a "conversational pace," sometimes referred to as the Rate of Perceived Exertion (RPE), to monitor your efforts during moderate activities, like walking. If you can talk and walk at the same time, you aren't working too hard. If you can sing and maintain your level of effort, you're probably not working hard enough. If you get out of breath quickly, you're probably working too hard – especially if you have to stop and catch your breath.

When should I use the target heart rate?

If you participate in more vigorous activities, like brisk walking and jogging, the "conversational pace" approach may not work. Try using the target heart rate. It works for many people, and is a good way for health professionals to monitor your progress.

The table below shows estimated target heart rates for different ages. Look for the age category closest to yours, and then read across to find your target heart rate.

Age	Target HR Zone 50–85 %	Average Maximum Heart Rate 100 %
20 years	100–170 beats per minute	200 beats per minute
25 years	98–166 beats per minute	195 beats per minute
30 years	95–162 beats per minute	190 beats per minute
35 years	93–157 beats per minute	185 beats per minute
40 years	90–153 beats per minute	180 beats per minute
45 years	88–149 beats per minute	175 beats per minute
50 years	85–145 beats per minute	170 beats per minute
55 years	83–140 beats per minute	165 beats per minute
60 years	80–136 beats per minute	160 beats per minute
65 years	78–132 beats per minute	155 beats per minute
70 years	75–128 beats per minute	150 beats per minute

Your maximum heart rate is about 220 minus your age. The figures above are averages, so use them as general guidelines.

Note: A few high blood pressure medications lower the maximum heart rate and thus the target zone rate. If you're taking such medicine, call your physician to find out if you need to use a lower target heart rate.

How should I pace myself?

When starting an exercise program, aim at the lowest part of your target zone (50 percent) during the first few weeks. Gradually build up to the higher part of your target zone (75 percent). After six months or more of regular exercise, you may be able to exercise comfortably at up to 85 percent of your maximum heart rate. However, you don't have to exercise that hard to stay in shape.

Training Zones

Healthy Heart Zone (Warm Up) — 50–60% of maximum heart rate. This is the easiest zone and probably the best zone for people just starting a fitness program. It can also be used as a warm up for more serious walkers. This zone has been shown to help lower body fat, blood pressure, and cholesterol. It also decreases the risk of degenerative diseases and has a low risk of injury. Of calories burned in this zone, 85% are fats!

Fitness Zone (Fat Burning) — 60–70% of maximum heart rate. This zone provides the same benefits as the healthy heart zone, but is more intense and burns more total calories. The percent of fat calories is still 85%.

Aerobic Zone (Endurance Training) — 70–80% of maximum heart rate. The aerobic zone will improve your cardiovascular and respiratory system AND increase the size and strength of your heart. This is the preferred zone if you are training for an endurance event. More calories are burned, with 50% being from fat.

Anaerobic Zone (Performance Training) — 80–90% of maximum heart rate. Benefits of this zone include an improved VO2 maximum (the highest amount of oxygen one can consume during exercise), and thus an improved cardio-respiratory system, and a higher lactate-tolerance ability, which means your endurance will improve and you'll be able to fight fatigue better. This is a high-intensity zone burning more calories, with 15% from fat.

Red Line (Maximum Effort) — 90–100% of maximum heart rate. Although this zone burns the highest number of calories/min, it is very intense. Most people can stay in this zone for only short periods. You should train in this zone only if you are in very good shape and have been cleared by a physician to do so.

Step Test

This test is designed to measure your cardiovascular endurance. Using a 12-inch-high bench (or a similar-sized stair in your house), step on and off for three minutes. Step up with one foot and then the other. Step down with one foot, followed by the other foot. Try to maintain a steady four-beat cycle. It's easy to maintain if you say, "Up, up, down, down." Go at a steady and consistent pace. At the end of three minutes, remain standing and immediately check your heart rate by taking your pulse for one minute.

This home step test is based on the Harvard Step Assessment. If you want to keep track of your cardiovascular improvements do this test four to six weeks after you start your exercise program and see if you have improved.

3-Minute Step Test (Men)

Age	18-25	26-35	36-45	46-55	56-65	65+
Excellent	<79	<81	<83	<87	<86	<88
Good	79-89	81-89	83-96	87-97	86-97	88-96
Above Average	90-99	90-99	97-103	98-105	98-103	97-103
Average	100-105	100-107	104-112	106-116	104-112	104-113
Below Average	106-116	108-117	113-119	117-122	113-120	114-120
Poor	117-128	118-128	120-130	123-132	121-129	121-130
Very Poor	>128	>128	>130	>132	>129	>130

3-Minute Step Test (Women)

Age	18-25	26-35	36-45	46-55	56-65	65+
Excellent	<85	<88	<90	<94	<95	<90
Good	85-98	88-99	90-102	94-104	95-104	90-102
Above Average	99-108	100-111	103-110	105-115	105-112	103-115
Average	109-117	112-119	111-118	116-120	113-118	116-122
Below Average	118-126	120-126	119-128	121-129	119-128	123-128
Poor	127-140	127-138	129-140	130-135	129-139	129-134

Very Poor	>140	>138	>140	>135	>139	>134

Push-Up Test

How many can you do? Men should use the standard military-style push-up position, with only the hands and the toes touching the floor. Women have the additional option of using the "bent knee" position. To do this, kneel on the floor, hands on either side of the chest, and keep your back straight. Do as many push-ups as possible until exhaustion. Count the total number of push-ups performed. Use the chart below to find out how you rate.

Push-Up Test (Men)

Age	17-19	20-29	30-39	40-49	50-59	60-65
Excellent	>56	>47	>41	>34	>31	>30
Good	47-56	39-47	34-41	28-34	25-31	24-30
Above Average	35-46	30-39	25-33	21-28	18-24	17-23
Average	19-34	17-29	13-24	11-20	9-17	6-16
Below Average	11-18	10-16	8-12	6-10	5-8	3-5
Poor	4-10	4-9	2-7	1-5	1-4	1-2
Very Poor	<4	<4	<2	0	0	0

Push-Up Test (Women)

Age	17-19	20-29	30-39	40-49	50-59	60-65
Excellent	>35	>36	>37	>31	>25	>23
Good	27-35	30-36	30-37	25-31	21-25	19-23
Above Average	21-27	23-29	22-30	18-24	15-20	13-18
Average	11-20	12-22	10-21	8-17	7-14	5-12

Below Average	6-10	7-11	5-9	4-7	3-6	2-4
Poor	2-5	2-6	1-4	1-3	1-2	1
Very Poor	0-1	0-1	0	0	0	0

Squat Test

How many squats can you do? Stand in front of a chair or bench with your feet at shoulder-width apart, facing away from it. Place your hands on your hips. Squat down and lightly touch the chair before standing up. A good-sized chair is one that makes your knees at right angles when you are sitting. Keep doing this until you're fatigued.

Squat Test (Men)

Age	18-25	26-35	36-45	46-55	56-65	65+
Excellent	>49	>45	>41	>35	>31	>28
Good	44-49	40-45	35-41	29-35	25-31	22-28
Above Average	39-43	35-39	30-34	25-38	21-24	19-21
Average	35-38	31-34	27-29	22-24	17-20	15-18
Below Average	31-34	29-30	23-26	18-21	13-16	11-14
Poor	25-30	22-28	17-22	13-17	9-12	7-10
Very Poor	<25	<22	<17	<9	<9	<7

Squat Test (Women)

Age	18-25	26-35	36-45	46-55	56-65	65+
Excellent	>43	>39	>33	>27	>24	>23
Good	37-43	33-39	27-33	22-27	18-24	17-23

Above Average	33-36	29-32	23-26	18-21	13-17	14-16
Average	29-32	25-28	19-22	14-17	10-12	11-13
Below Average	25-28	21-24	15-18	10-13	7-9	5-10
Poor	18-24	13-20	7-14	5-9	3-6	2-4
Very Poor	<18	<20	<7	<5	<3	<2

Sit-Ups

Abdominal muscle strength and endurance are important for core stability and back support. This sit-up test measures the strength and endurance of the abdominals and hip-flexor muscles. Count how many you can do in one minute and then check the chart below for your rating.

Starting Position: Lie on a carpeted or cushioned floor, with your knees bent at approximately right angles and your feet flat on the ground. Your hands should be resting on your thighs.

Technique: Squeeze your stomach, push your back flat, and raise high enough for your hands to slide along your thighs to touch the tops of your knees. Don't pull with your neck or head, and keep your lower back on the floor. Return to the starting position.

1-Minute Sit-Up Test (Men)

Age	18-25	26-35	36-45	46-55	56-65	65+
Excellent	>49	>45	>41	>35	>31	>28
Good	44-49	40-45	35-41	29-35	25-31	22-28
Above Average	39-43	35-39	30-34	25-28	21-24	19-21
Average	35-38	31-34	27-29	22-24	17-20	15-18
Below Average	31-34	29-30	23-26	18-21	13-16	11-14
Poor	25-30	22-28	17-22	13-17	9-12	7-10

Very Poor	<25	<22	<17	<9	<9	<7

1-Minute Sit-Up Test (Women)

Age	18-25	26-35	36-45	46-55	56-65	65+
Excellent	>43	>39	>33	>27	>24	>23
Good	37-43	33-39	27-33	22-27	18-24	17-23
Above Average	33-36	29-32	23-26	18-21	13-17	14-16
Average	29-32	25-28	19-22	14-17	10-12	11-13
Below Average	25-28	21-24	15-18	10-13	7-9	5-10
Poor	18-24	13-20	7-14	5-9	3-6	2-4
Very Poor	<18	<20	<7	<5	<3	<2

Source: adapted from Golding, et al. (1986). *The Y's way to physical fitness* (3rd ed.)

This Will Only Hurt a Little... Finding Out Your Body Fat Percentage

Body Composition

Body composition is simply the ratio of lean body mass to fat body mass. Too much fat can lead to health problems like heart disease, diabetes, high cholesterol, and other serious conditions. If you keep your body fat within a reasonable level, you'll be healthier and, of course, slimmer.

For women, a body fat of 10–12% is essential, 14–20% is considered a healthy range for athletes, 21–24% is healthy for fitness, 25–31% is considered an "acceptable" range, and anything above 32% is considered obese. For men, 2–4% body fat is essential, 6–13% is an athletic body fat range, 14–17% is considered a "fit" range, 18–25% is acceptable, and anything above 26% is considered obese. So, how do you find out what your body fat is?

Below are the most popular methods for testing body composition.

Common Methods Used to Find the Fat Percentage

Calipers

This method uses calipers to measure skin fold thickness at several areas of your body.

How it works: A trainer pinches your skin at different areas and measures them with calipers. Results are plugged into a formula to determine your body fat.

Have you been pinched lately? Maybe you haven't, but you've probably heard people talking about how low their body fat is.

"Great, I have six percent body fat." Not so fast, just ask a different trainer to measure your body fat, and suddenly you have sixteen percent? The problem is there is a great deal of human error when using calipers. What would seem like a small difference in measurement can make a big difference to your overall percentage. There are many variables that affect your percentage: gender, ethnicity, fitness level, and age. The accuracy of body fat calipers is rated within 4% if you have an experienced trainer administering the test, so take it with a grain of low-sodium salt.

Hydrostatic Weighing

This is just a fancy way of saying underwater weighing. This test is one of the more accurate ones.

How it works:

You sit on a scale inside a tank of water and blow out as much air as you can. You are dunked underwater, where you blow out even more air. Since fat is lighter than water, the more fat you have, the more you'll float. The scale measures underwater weight to figure out body density. The margin of error is around 2–3%, but the accuracy depends on the amount of air you expel. You have to blow it all out or it won't be as accurate.

This is a difficult way to measure body fat, since it can be uncomfortable and even scary to be dunked underwater with no air in the old lungs. If you want to use hydrostatic weighing make sure you don't pay too much at an overpriced "Health Spa," some universities offer this test for around \$25–\$50.

Bioelectrical Impedance

I prefer this method above all others because it's quick, easy and the scales can be obtained at a variety of stores including pharmacies, department stores as well as specialty stores like *The Sharper Image* and *GNC*.

The basic principle of bioelectrical impedance is this: As you stand on the scale a signal passes from your feet; the faster the signal travels, the more muscle you have. The results are based on the fact that water conducts electricity. Fat contains almost no water, while muscle is about 70% water.

Depending on the brand of the scale, this method can be accurate within the 4% margin of error the calipers have, but the results are affected by hydration, food intake, and skin temperature. If you're dehydrated, your body fat percentage will read higher than it is. This is an easy way to test your body fat. Be sure to test it at the same time of day.

The Exercise Program

Choose Your Primary Aerobic Device

- Treadmill

- Bicycle

- Elliptical or stepper

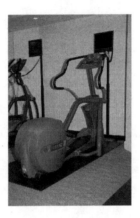

- Do It Anywhere Cardio

- Ashley's *"Burn 'N Firm"* – Total Fitness DVD Series

Of the first three, my personal preference is the treadmill because for most people it's a device that's easy to use and has a history of success. Also, it's easy for me to get motivated to increase my pace when I combine it with some good, upbeat music and a mirror to encourage my progress.

For some (particularly if you are 30 or more pounds overweight), it may be preferable to begin with a bike, elliptical, stepper/climber or walking on an inclined treadmill.

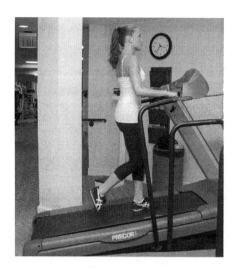

The reason is that jogging can put considerable stress on the back and joints, particularly the knees – and the last thing you need is an injury!

Your choice will depend on your personal preferences and understanding of your limitations, in consultation with your physician. Whichever you choose, START OFF SLOW and ADVANCE SLOWLY. Duration is more important than intensity.

Hey! Excuse me! No disrespect to the doctor, but if you want a really simple, fun, and effective exercise routine that incorporates all the components of our Dump Your Trainer Fitness Program, check out my "Burn 'N Firm" exercise DVD. More about it later.

The 80/20 Rule

If you're to achieve your goal of weight loss, you need to focus on the exercises that burn calories while also toning the muscles in the process. This is exactly the opposite of what you get with a trainer. In fact, recently some well-connected "celebrity" gurus have been advocating various "cardio-free" exercise and diet programs, with as little as one hour per week of strictly resistance training. Alternatively, a trainer may tell you to get aerobic exercise on your own time. But let's be realistic – who has any more time?

I have no intention of wasting time disputing the ridiculous logic of the "cardio-free" programs. Suffice it to say that the epidemic of obesity in this country is certainly not the result of an excess of cardio-intensive exercise. In fact, there is overwhelming evidence indicating that it's most likely a direct consequence of the lack of it. Furthermore, according to a study in the "Journal of Gerontology: Medical Sciences" and reported in "The Wall Street Journal," as little as three hours of aerobic exercise per week can reverse the brain shrinkage which normally starts in a person's 40's and actually lead to regeneration of new brain cells - a phenomenon which had previously been considered impossible. Strength training and stretching had no effect whatsoever. In addition, recent studies have also demonstrated that regular aerobic exercise can actually reverse earlier radiological findings of pathology in the coronary arteries.

On the other hand, a solid resistive/toning component can be a great adjunct to an overall fitness program. As pointed out in a recent article by Dr. Mark Williams, et al., in the journal *Circulation*, some of the potential benefits may include "enhanced cardiovascular health, weight management, and prevention of disability..." The researchers further note that: "Incorporating resistance training in the training regimen can potentially improve maintenance of interest and compliance." But they also add this qualification: "Because of the extensive evidence supporting the benefits of aerobic exercise training on modulating cardiovascular risk factors…resistance training should be used as a complement to, and not a replacement for, aerobic exercise."

My personal recommendation is: Get your 70–80% aerobic exercise first, and then get your 15–20% muscle strengthening later at the gym, on your own or, if you prefer, with a trainer.

I find that if I do my jogging first thing in the morning, then I'm able to get in the strengthening later during the day or evening. It's far easier to find 10–20 minutes for muscle strengthening than it is to get motivated for 40–60 minutes of jogging after a hard and perhaps stressful day.

For optimum results, I recommend a program of 40–60 minutes of aerobic exercise (including the warm up) first thing in the morning, and then another 20 minutes (perhaps on an alternate device, such as a bike) in the evening, ideally along with an additional 20 minutes of strengthening. If you follow this program, in addition to the dietary recommendations, your results will be extraordinary.

Time of Day – Right Away

There are experts who would debate this point until all the celebrities get out of rehab. Some say you burn more at night, others say in the morning, others say some combination of both. Forget this argument. From a practical standpoint, it's all just a bunch of meaningless noise.

What you need to do is get your aerobic exercise every day, and the best way to ensure this is to do it first thing in the morning, before anything else can distract you.

I used to have to be at the clinic by 6:30 a.m. That meant getting up at 4:00 a.m. to get my exercise in. Every day I woke up, I hated myself. I fought myself, I cursed myself. But 50 lbs. later, I loved myself. You will, too.

So calculate one hour for exercise before you do anything else and set the clock an hour earlier, if that is what it takes. And, allow no excuses from yourself. Morning exercise is your new religion.

Stretching

Pay particular attention to stretching the leg muscles, especially the calf and thigh. Stretching the calf muscles is particularly important if you're jogging. Nothing will lay you up quicker than a cramped or strained gastrocnemius muscle. So make sure you stretch for at least two to five minutes before beginning your run. Make sure to use steady, slow stretching and avoid bouncing.

I often watch someone hop off the treadmill at the gym, rush to the shower, or jump in the car, without even a quick cool down or stretch. Great, you just ran three miles, but you may not be feeling so good tomorrow or the next day if you don't take the time to stretch out the muscles you've just worked. The keys to preventing injuries are warming up, cooling down, and stretching.

The key to proper stretching lies in the way you perform the exercise. When you're stretching certain parts of your body, you should not feel pain. Staying relaxed is very important to stretching properly. Make sure your body is not tight. Go slow! Always stretch slowly and evenly. Hold the stretch for about fifteen seconds and release slowly, as well. Never bounce or jerk while stretching. This can cause injury as a muscle is pushed beyond its ability. All stretches should be smooth and slow. Don't forget to breathe. Flexibility exercises should be relaxing. Deep, easy, even breathing is key to relaxation. Never hold your breath while you stretch. Your shoulders, hands, and feet should be kept relaxed as you stretch.

Here are some basic stretches you should do daily.

Hamstrings: Sit on the floor with one leg straight in front of you and the other leg bent (with the sole of the foot touching the inside thigh of the outstretched leg). Keep your back straight and lean forward from the hips. Slide your arms forward toward your outstretched foot. Stop when you feel a pull in the hamstring. Hold for 15 seconds. Repeat with the other leg extended.

Hips: Lie on your back. Bend your left leg and bring it toward you. Grasp your left knee gently with your right hand and pull it slightly down and to the right until you feel a stretch. Turn your head to the left. Your right leg should stay flat on the floor. Hold for 10 seconds. Repeat with the other leg.

Lower back: Lay flat on the floor with knees bent. Use your hands to pull them toward your chest. Lift your head and shoulders off the floor until your head is approximately six inches from your knees. Cross your ankles. Gently rock yourself back and forth in this position for 30 seconds.

Quadriceps: Lie on your right side with your right knee bent at a 90-degree angle. Bend your left leg and hold on to the ankle with your left hand. Gently pull your left heel in toward the left side of your butt. As soon as you feel a stretch in your left quad, slowly lower your left knee toward the floor, behind your right knee. Hold for 15 seconds. Repeat with the other leg.

Calves: Stand at arm's length away from a wall, with your feet shoulder-width apart. Slide your left foot back approximately 18 inches, keeping the knee straight and both heels flat on the floor. Bend your right knee and slowly move your pelvis forward until you feel a stretch in the calf and Achilles tendon of the left leg. Hold for 15 seconds. Repeat with the other leg.

Warming Up

Stretching will help you warm up a bit, but it is most important to start your exercise very slowly. Don't start out at a jog or pumping the bike or stepper. Let the blood begin to flow gradually by getting started slowly and moving up steadily to your workout level.

Step Up – Step Down

Start slowly. If you're doing the morning routine, then you'll probably still be half asleep and this shouldn't be a problem. Increase your pace in small increments (as explained later in the book) to a maximum comfortable exercise range, then decrease in regular intervals.

Finish off walking until your heart rate returns to normal. A pounding heart will force blood into the leg veins, and if the leg muscles are not pumping it back, the blood will collect there, potentially leading to vascular damage and varicose veins.

Sample Programs:
For illustration, here is an example for a person in good health, with no physical restrictions, looking to lose 20 lbs. and using the treadmill.

Step Up
Start your warm up at 2.5 miles/hour for one minute. Increase to 3.0 miles/hour for two minutes, then increase to 3.5 miles/hour for two minutes. Next, increase your pace to jogging at 4.0 miles/hour for five minutes. Accelerate 0.5 miles/hour every five minutes, to a maximum speed that you can maintain comfortably for five minutes. *Do not overdue it!* Contrary to the "no pain, no gain" philosophies espoused by the popular, media hyped, 'fitness' shows, pushing yourself too far can put a quick end to your program through injuries as well as permanent damage to

your joints, spine and cardiovascular system. Ignore these programs. They're not really concerned about your health - only improving their TV ratings.

Step Down

This is a very important component, since here is where you'll greatly increase the total number of calories burned without stressing or straining yourself. From your maximum pace, decrease your speed 0.5 miles/hour for one to five minutes (depending on tolerance). Continue to decrease your pace 0.5 miles/hour every one to five minutes until you return to the 3.5 miles/hour pace, at which you'll be back to walking. Decrease your walking pace by 0.5 miles/hour every one to two minutes until you return to 2.5 miles/hour.

Continue this pace until your heart rate returns to near normal. Note the calories that you burned. By adding the step down component, you will have burned an additional 10–20% beyond what you would have burned on a typical step up program alone. Over time, this will make a huge difference in how quickly you'll lose those extra pounds.

Motivation

Many people say they need a trainer to provide them with motivation. What they're really saying is that they're looking at their exercise program as a social alternative. Working with a trainer can be very social. At the rates they charge, they will be very conversant, understanding, and pleasant. Unfortunately, this won't help you lose those extra pounds that would truly help improve your social life.

Instead, think about the following methods to motivate you in a more rewarding aerobic program. Furthermore, consider participating in some team sports or dancing programs, as mentioned later on.

Dump the TV – Turn on the Music

Let's face it: It's all about motivation. Television motivates you to sit around, not to exercise. It certainly won't motivate you to increase your pace during exercise. Nothing motivates like music with a beat. So turn off the TV and turn on the music. You'll see a dramatic increase in your motivation during exercise and will lose those extra pounds much faster.

Of course, there are exceptions. A friend of mine gets his motivation for cycling by watching the Playboy Channel. Hey, to each his own. Others get upbeat watching BET or other music video channels. Whatever works! But don't expect to get motivated by watching soaps or *Oprah* during your exercise. It's more likely that they'll keep your pace to a minimum.

The Beauty of Mirrors

Let your narcissistic qualities work for you. Don't hide in denial. Put a full-length mirror in front of your treadmill/stepper/bike/dance space. Accept what you look like now and plan what you're going to look like later. A touch of reality will go a long way to motivating you in your weight loss program. In the beginning and over time, the facts will speak for themselves and you'll slowly see the results as you witness the metamorphosis.

Dance, Dance, Dance

In front of the mirror by yourself, in a class, or out on the town. Better yet, all of the above. It's fun, social, and great exercise. It can also be invigorating, so make sure you're not overdoing the intensity. Remember, it's exercise and you need to follow the rules for aerobic exercise in general.

One caution: ADD IT TO YOUR AEROBIC PROGRAM, BUT DON'T USE IT AS A SUBSTITUTE until you can establish a regular routine. You can burn an additional 200–400 calories per dance session, or 600–800 calories per aerobics dance class – which, combined with your basic workout, will accelerate you to your goal. (See our Cardio Dance section later in the book for further insight and information.)

Weights/Resistance Training

Tone, don't bulk!
If your goal is to look like the Incredible Hulk then you're reading the wrong book. This program is designed for those who want to look lean and sexy, not buffed and intimidating.

My emphasis is to show you how to increase muscle tone and strength to support improved conditioning. Unless you plan to be a bodybuilder or furniture mover, forget the bulk. It won't help your health.

There's a lot of disagreement in the exercise community as to which is better: free weights, machines, or other weight-lifting methods. Again, from your standpoint it's all noise. Choose the resistance method you like best. Resistance bands, free weights, machines or simply using your own body weight will all get the job done.

For now, focus on working multiple muscle groups at light to moderate resistance, with more emphasis on repetitions. You should be able to comfortably do 10–15 repetitions without straining. Again, the key issue is not to injure yourself. Nothing will destroy your program quicker than injury.

For the novice weight lifter or newly activated former athlete, I prefer using the machines. Their responses are more controlled, and the risk of straining and injury should be lower.

There is also disagreement among the gurus as to how many sets should be done for each muscle groups, and which groups should be done in various orders and regimens. Whether you want to do two or three sets of certain machines or one set of every machine, the important point is that you do what you feel like doing on any particular day and not strain yourself doing so. I have to admit to some bias in doing one set of each of the different machines available. The logic is that you still get your exercise, but also tone a greater variety of muscles than you might otherwise. In any case, focus on the reps and put less emphasis on the weight.

For the initial prescription of resistance training, Dr. Williams and the researchers with the American Heart Association (AHA) recommend that "it should be performed in a rhythmic manner at a moderate to slow controlled speed. It should encompass a full range of motion. Breath-holding and straining (Valsalva maneuver) should be avoided by exhaling during the contraction or exertion phase of the lift and inhaling during the relaxation phase."

The researchers further state: "In addition, resistance training should alternate between upper and lower body work, allowing adequate rest between exercises. The initial weight load should not exceed 8 to 12 repetitions per set for healthy sedentary adults or 10 to 15 repetitions at a low level of resistance (e.g., less than 40% of 1-repetition maximum) for older individuals (aged > 50 to 60 years), more frail persons, or cardiac patients."

They further point out that: "At first, resistance training should not exceed a single set performed 2 days/week. It should involve the major muscle groups of the upper and lower extremities. Suitable exercises include chest press, shoulder press, triceps extension, biceps curl, pull-down (upper back), lower-back extension, abdominal crunch/curl-up, quadriceps extension or leg press, leg curls (hamstrings), and calf raise."

One last note: This is the one area of the exercise program that may justify a competent trainer. Just make sure that it takes up no more than 20% of your total program time and does not eat into the more important 80% cardio/aerobic workout.

Strength in Numbers?

Workout Buddies

Having someone to workout with seems like an obvious advantage. Unfortunately, relying on someone else to maintain your program can be inherently self-destructive. My advice is to build your program without any outside dependence or influence. If a buddy ends up coming along sometimes (or always), great – but don't make that person's participation a requisite to your program, or you risk turning their half-hearted motivation into excuses for breaking your own routine.

This is particularly important for the morning component. Let's face it, getting out of bed early every day is going to be hard enough to do yourself. Don't even think about expecting any other "fool" to join your "new religion." Keep the faith and save your own "soul" first. You can work on the rest of humanity later.

Even for the afternoon/evening component, my suggestion is that you have your buddy meet you at the gym (or other location), not go together. This way their excuses will not affect you. If they actually do show up, fine. My expectation is that 70% of the time they won't. Don't worry. Once they see how great you're looking, they'll follow.

Bottom line: Don't let your workout depend on anyone other than yourself. If you'd like to work out with your buddy, have your buddy join you. Or join a cardio class and make new buddies who are also dedicated to improving their health.

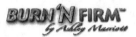

Don't have a treadmill? Can't or don't want to jog around the block? Want to alternate your exercise program each day?

Ashley Marriott's 'Burn 'N Firm' program is an exhilarating blend of kickboxing, body firming and dance techniques, including Latin, Disco and Cardio. Get the sizzle of South Beach with the heart pumpin' body groovin' feel of hottest workouts!

You can order directly via the web at: www.burnnfirm.com or www.DumpYourTrainer.com

Getting Started

You should review the following program outlines and guidelines so that you have a general understanding of the program and where you fit in. Later on, we'll provide you with a day-by-day program that you can follow in detail. In the appendices, we'll also provide you with an easy-to-follow check sheet that you can copy and use during your journey to fitness.

Control Your Environment – At-Home Preparation

First, take a few minutes and eliminate temptation at home. Clear out all the junk food from your cupboards.

After you review the meal plan, stock up on the recommended ingredients to create healthy meals and snacks.

You've already taken the first step to fitness success. Each day, week, and month you'll build on this success to achieve your goals!

You should plan on a 30 - 40 minute morning exercise program and a 30 - 40 minute evening program. Over time, this should be increased to 40 - 60 minutes in the morning and 40 minutes or more in the evening, as your endurance and conditioning improves.

Evaluate Where You Stand

After assessing your overall health with your doctor, and taking into account any limitations he or she has advised you of, begin by assessing where you stand based on your weight.

What follows is a general outline of the program details based loosely on your current and progress weight. Of course, you, in conjunction with your physician, should modify these according to your particular situation.

Group #1: I'm 5–20 pounds overweight

Morning:
Begin the first week with 10 minutes of walking, followed by 10 minutes of jogging and 10 minutes of walking, then progress slowly and gradually from there.

Evening:
Begin with 10 minutes of walking on the treadmill, or 10 minutes on the bike or elliptical. Follow with 20 minutes of toning on the weight machines. Increase to walking and jogging or increase pace slowly over time. After the first week, you can try a beginner aerobic dance or cardio class, with caution and without pushing yourself to keep up. Proceed as tolerated.

Group #2: I'm 20–40 pounds overweight

Morning:
Begin with 20 minutes of walking and five minutes of slow jogging, and progress very slowly from there. By the end of Phase 1 (Day 21), you should be able to increase your pace to that of Group #1.

Evening:
Begin with 10 minutes of walking on the treadmill, or 10 minutes on the bike or elliptical. Follow with 20 minutes of toning on the weight machines. Increase to walking and jogging or increase pace slowly over time.

Group #3: I'm 40–60 pounds overweight

Morning:
Begin walking 20–30 minutes and gradually increase your pace over the next 20 days. By Day 13, you may be able to walk for 15 minutes, jog for five minutes, and walk for five minutes more. By the end of Phase 1, you may be able to move on to Group #2.

Evening:

Begin with 10 minutes of walking on the treadmill, or 10 minutes on the bike or elliptical. Follow with 20 minutes of toning on the weight machines. Increase the pace slowly over time.

Group #4: I'm more than 60 pounds overweight

Morning:

Jogging should be avoided since it may cause damage to the spine, hips, and knees. It's best to combine walking and riding a stationary/semi-recumbent bicycle until ready to move on to Group #3. Start with walking for 20 minutes, and then a slow to moderate pace on the bicycle for 10 minutes.

Evening:

Begin with 10 minutes of walking on the treadmill, or 10 minutes on the bike or elliptical. Follow with 20 minutes of toning on the weight machines. Increase your walking pace slowly over time.

Detailed Starting Exercise Program – Example

Morning Program

This example will assume that you're using a home treadmill for your morning workout and that you're 20–40 pounds overweight. If you don't have a treadmill, going around the block repeatedly will suffice; just make sure you have running shoes with excellent cushioning. Alternatively, you can just follow the program in Ashley's "Burn 'N Firm" – Total Fitness DVD right in your own home.

In either case, to adjust the program to your own circumstances, follow the above guidelines according to your group.

If you work, you'll need to get up an hour earlier in the morning. What! Are you out of your mind? Sorry, yes, you heard me right – and yes, you'll curse me and yourself every morning. Just do it! When I was in practice, I had to be at work at 6:30 every morning. This meant getting up at 4:00 a.m. Boy, was I pissed… but every day the scale went down, and 50 pounds later nobody could even recognize me and I felt great!

If you're a "stay at home" parent or worker, then you don't need to get up earlier – but you do need to get you workout in before anything else (other than getting the kids off to wherever). Don't start anything. No phone calls. No housework. Nothing. If you do, then you'll never get to your workout, guaranteed. If you don't adhere to this simple principle, then your weight loss program is doomed from the start.

After taking care of nature's needs, begin some slow stretches, especially of the gastrocnemius muscle (back of your lower leg) and the Achilles tendon region. Don't bounce – just slow tension. Stretch and relax the muscles until they loosen up.

Get on the treadmill and start to walk at 2.5 miles per hour for one minute, and then increase the pace to 3.0 miles per hour for two minutes. You should be starting to wake up now, though still groaning a bit at yourself in the mirror.

After two minutes, increase the pace to 3.5 miles per hour for another two minutes.

Now you can increase the pace to 4.0 miles per hour and do some very casual jogging for five minutes.

After five minutes, you'll increase your pace to 4.5 miles per hour for five more minutes. You may be tempted to increase your pace even more, now that you're awake and feeling good – but don't, at least not for the first week or two. Remember, injuries are your worst enemy and getting overly enthusiastic during the early phase will certainly lead to program-stopping injuries and pain. After the first two to three weeks, you can slowly and progressively increase your pace, but never to the point at which it leaves you in pain.

This is the important part. Make sure you do it every time you work out. It's called the step down segment, and will result in your burning an extra 10–20% more calories – almost effortlessly. Drop the pace down to 4.0 miles per hour for another minute of jogging, and then after a minute down to 3.5 miles per hour for another minute more of brisk walking. Do the same the following minute by dropping the pace down to 3.0 miles per hour, and then in a minute down to 2.5. After a minute, you're done.

Good work! You're awake. You feel great and you're on your way. Not so bad, huh? Well, except for the waking up early part. Sorry, but you'll probably never really like that. Deal with it!

Detailed Evening and Toning Program

Aerobic Component
This module will assume that you're in Group #2, including an evening workout, and that you're working out at a local gym.

Arrive at the gym and begin with a five-minute warm up on either a bicycle or elliptical, if available.

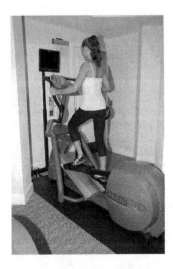

Move over to a treadmill and make sure you again stretch out those gastrocs, etc.

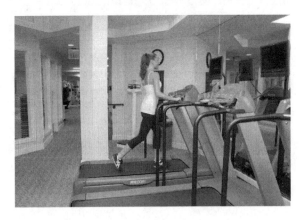

Begin the step up component as in the morning exercise, and increase your pace in increments until you're jogging at 4.0–4.5 miles per hour for five-minute segments again.

Begin the step down sequence and decrease your pace at the same rate as the morning program.

Congratulations! The aerobic component is done.

Toning Component

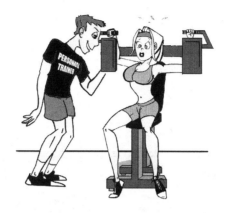

"I think we should focus on your upper body."

I'm always asked what my philosophy is regarding free weights vs. machines, the ideal number of repetitions and sets, and if working selected muscle groups on different days will maximize a person's workout program. My answer is always the same: Give me a ____ break! You're not preparing for the Olympics.

Maybe (and that's a definite maybe) this type of "science" has meaning to a competitive athlete, but to you it should be just more meaningless noise. What you need to be focusing on is getting through your workout as simply as possible, so that you lose weight while toning as many of the muscle groups as you can. Start out with 10–12 reps at a comfortable weight load. If you find that you can do 12 reps easily, consider either increasing the reps to 15 or increasing the weight load to the point at which you can do 10 reps <u>without straining</u>.

What follows is a simple example that should tone all the major muscle groups and give you an overall sense of balanced toning. You should be able to accomplish this at most gyms. Furthermore, most of the exercises work overlapping muscle groups, so in effect you will be doing multiple sets anyway.

Note: Every gym is laid out differently, so modify your routine to go conveniently from one machine to the next. Just try to work opposing or different muscle groups at each stop. For example, bicep curls followed by triceps presses or rotational abdominal twists, etc.

After your cool down and drink a few sips of water, move to the floor or slant board for some crunches. Again, don't push it. The last thing you need is an injury. One more thing: if you get to a machine and it's being used, just move on to the next exercise and come back to it later or on another day. There's plenty of overlap already built into the program. Just keep moving.

Do a set of 10–20 crunches and move on.

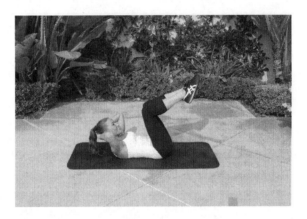

Now move on to the overhead press machine and do 10–12 presses, using weights that don't cause you to strain even on your last press.

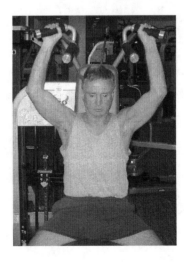

Next move on to the biceps curling machine and again do 10–12 curls without straining at all.

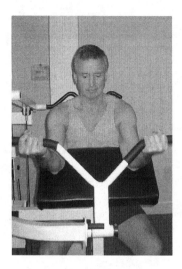

Next move on to 10 – 12 reps of triceps extension.

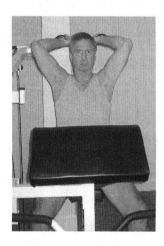

Move on to the deltoid lift and do 10–12 lifts. Again, no straining.

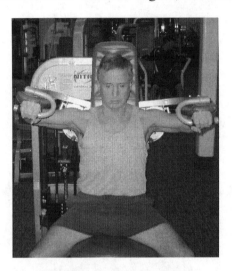

Crunch machine for 10–12 crunches.

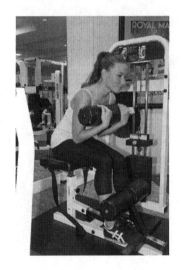

Now add some pectoral flies for 10–12 reps.

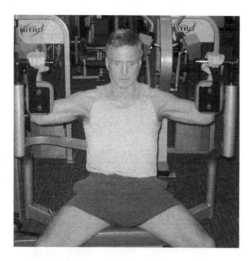

Move on to the forward press for 10–12 reps.

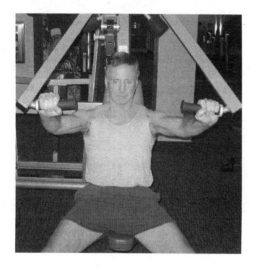

Rotational weighted (go light at first) abdominals for 10–12 reps.

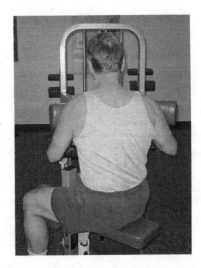

Angled forward press for 10–12 reps guided free weights or slanted bench machine.

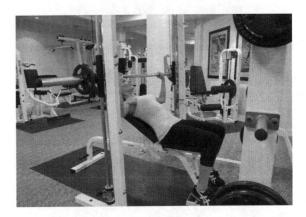

At this point, I like to throw in a bit of light free-weight curls for 10–12 reps, since it's hard to find a really good curling machine. (Note: you've now done a second set of curls using different equipment.)

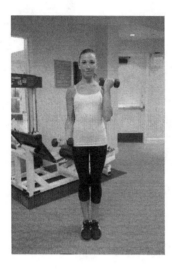

Now move over to the lumbar (lower) back extension device for 5–8 reps.

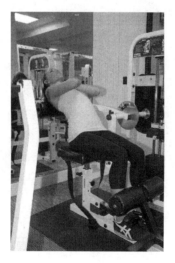

On to the full extension fly machine (if your gym has one).

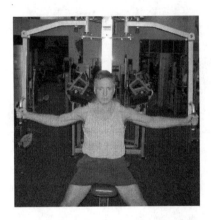 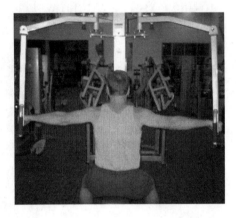

Do 10–12 forward fly reps to work those pectorals (chest), and then turn around, decrease the weight by half, and do 10–12 backward fly's for the upper back.

Now move over to the overhead pull to work the latissimus dorsi muscles for 10–12 reps.

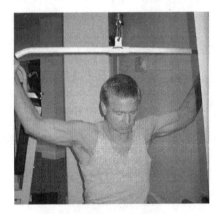

Move over to the upper back machine and do 10–12 pulls. Again, no straining.

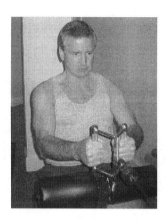

You're done.

You've just completed an aerobic workout and overall toning of most of the major muscle groups. In time, you'll start to feel sleek all over!

Wait! What about the legs?

I have to admit that here is where I perhaps cheat a bit – at least during the early phase of the program. It's not that I don't think that toning the legs is a good idea. It's just that 80% of the program already works the legs, and the notion that these exercises will localize the fat loss to the legs is false.

If you would like to add them, certainly do, but do so very cautiously and after the second or third week of the program. Overworking these areas can really tighten the muscles and make it very difficult to continue the aerobic component. If time is a factor, my suggestion is to add in these exercises on alternate days.

Ladies, if you want to really tone up those butts and thighs while reducing the appearance of cellulite then check out my stability ball exercise chapter.

Start with very light weights and a 10–12 rep set of leg flexions, extensions and gluteus presses.

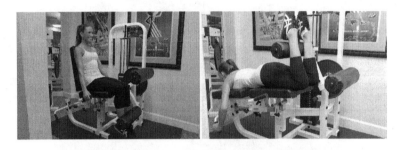

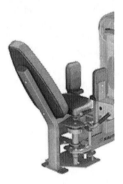

In addition, you can throw in some abductions and adductions for 10–12 reps.

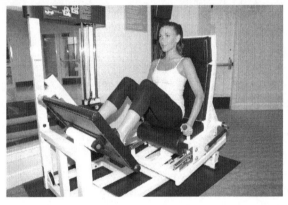

Now Smile!

You've just completed a full aerobic and toning workout without having wasted a dime on a Personal Trainer.

No Gym Membership – No Problem

You can get an excellent resistance-training workout at home, with or without any equipment. I guarantee everyone has at least one piece of resistance equipment already – YOU! Your own body weight provides excellent resistance. Think of a push-up; many top trainers regard this as a near-perfect exercise. Take a look around – what other things are already in your house, like stairs, a chair, or water jugs? Be creative. I often train clients at their homes, and some of them do have beautifully equipped home gyms, but I also train people with nothing but the little bag of tricks I bring with me – a stability ball and a set of resistance bands. Guess what? The fancy equipment doesn't make the difference – it is the energy, form, and focus you put into it.

There are tons of options if you want to create an at-home gym, and if you have the money, I say go for it. I see many benefits of training at home:

Nobody cares what you look like (you can work out in your pj's).

No wasted time driving to and from the gym.

No waiting in line to use sweaty equipment.

No excuses that the gym is closed – if you're up at 3 a.m., you can do it then.

But before you go out and spend a lot of money on fancy gym equipment, you may want to start slowly and make sure you really need it. I'd hate to have you using that $1,500 Bowflex as a clothes hanger.

For less than $50, you can get two of my favorite training tools: a resistance band and a stability ball. That's less than a month's membership at many health clubs. Most of the resistance band sets and stability balls even come with workout posters, and some include an instructional DVD.

Why Resistance Bands?

Bands are great because they are cheap, compact, portable and versatile.

Because resistance bands are so compact and lightweight, you can easily take them along when you travel or if you want to sneak in a mini "at workout". Resistance bands generally come in three or four different levels of resistance and cost about $15 per band.

Yellow (thin)

Red (medium)

Green (heavy)

Blue (extra heavy)

Resistance Band Exercises

Beginners 2 sets of 12 repetitions of each exercise

Intermediate- 3 sets of 12 repetitions

Advanced- 3 sets of 15 repetitions

Remember you need to warm up first with 5-10 minutes of light aerobic exercise and stretch after.

Breathing: People tend to hold their breath when they are doing resistance exercise, which can be dangerous. Breathing is very important during exercise.

Exhale fully on the exertion phase of the lift. The exertion phase is the hardest part.

Inhale deeply on the easier phase, the release or the return to the starting position.

84

Resistance Band Squats

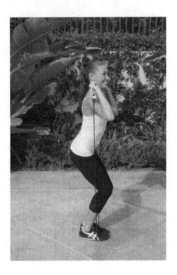 *Great exercise to get ready for sky season!*

Start by stepping on the resistance band with both feet.

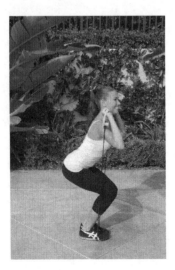

Try to use a shoulder width stance if you can.

Hold the resistance band at shoulder level with both hands. Start into a full squat while holding the band at shoulder height.

Return to the starting position and repeat.

Alternating Chest Press

Wrap the band around a sturdy object behind you at chest level.

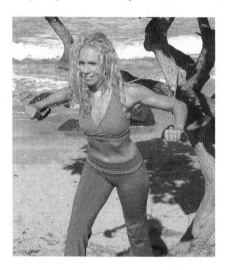

Secure band around a pole, tree or post. Stand with back to tree, feet slightly more than shoulder-width apart. Holding handles of band, extend both arms forward.

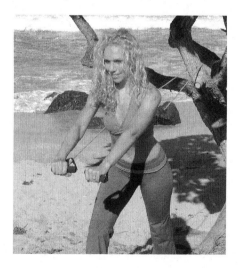

Holding handles of band, extend both arms forward. Then alternate chest press. Keep the right arm stationary and press the left arm out. Bring the left arm back and then press forward with the right arm.

Lat Pull

Stand with feet shoulder-width apart, holding a band securely underneath the feet. Hold one end of band in each hand. Lean forward at the waist so torso is parallel to the floor, arms bent 90 degrees.

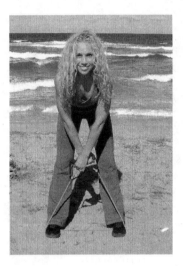

Contract the back and pull the band out while bringing the elbows towards the sky.

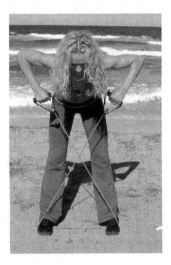

Return to start position.

Biceps Curls with Resistance Band

Stand with feet shoulder width apart, knees slightly bent, and at a staggered stance.

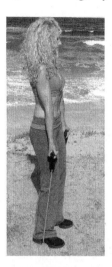

Step onto middle of tubing with back foot or both feet. Grasp ends with underhand grip with arms hanging down at sides. Elbows should be close to sides.

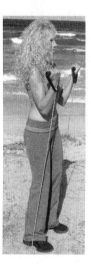

Flex at the elbows and curl band up to approximately shoulder level. Keep elbows close to sides throughout movement.

Return to start position.

Triceps Extension with Resistance Band

Secure band around a pole, tree or post. Start by holding the handles in both hands. Lean forward at waist, keeping back straight. Pull the band towards your hips, as if you were paddling on a surf board.

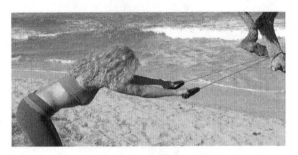

Extend from your elbow until your arm is fully extended.

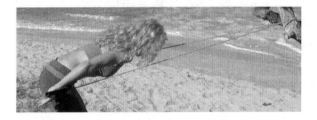

Return to the start position.

Resistance Band Single Arm Rows

Start by placing the band under one foot and stepping backwards with the other foot. Bend over keeping your back flat at a 45-degree angle.

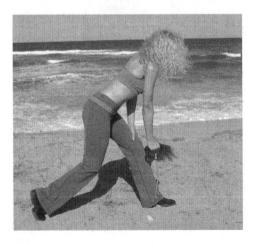

Pull the bands up towards your waist keeping your elbows in close together.

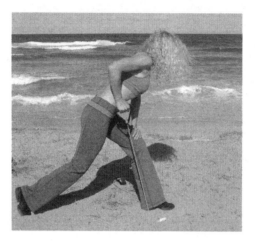

Squeeze your shoulder blades together when performing rowing motion.

Return to start position.

Standing Rows with Resistance Band

Secure band around a sturdy object.

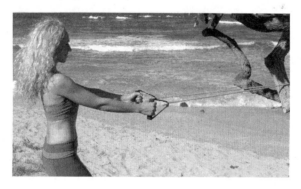

Secure band around a pole, tree or post. Start position: Grasp ends with a neutral grip (palms facing each other).

Raise band to side of body at shoulder height keeping elbows slightly bent.

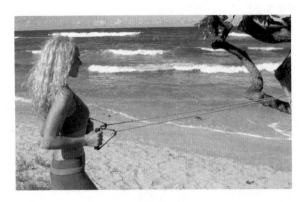

Slowly pull the bands to your hips. Return to start.

Torso Twist

Secure band around a pole, tree or post. Turn your upper body away from the object by twisting, without moving the legs.

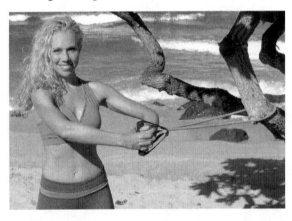

Return to starting position. Repeat on opposite side.

Band Assisted Stretching

Hamstring Stretch

Lie on the floor and loop band around the right foot, grabbing onto the bands to create tension.

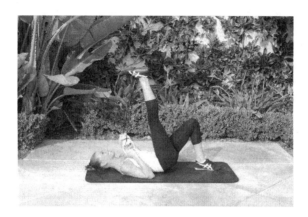

Straighten the right leg as much as you comfortably can while keeping the left leg bent on the floor. Gently pull the right leg towards you, stretching the back of the leg. Hold for 15-30 seconds and switch sides.

Upper Back Stretch

Sit on the floor with legs extended and loop the band around both feet. Cross the band and grab on to each side with both hands close to the feet.

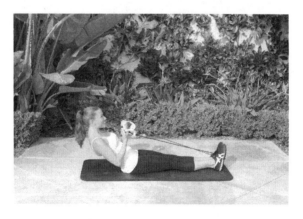

Gently curl the back, stretching it towards the back of the room and using the bands to create tension and add to the stretch. Keep the abs contracted and try not to collapse over the legs. Hold for 15-30 seconds.

Stability Ball

(Swiss, Balance, Stretch, and Physio Ball)
I don't care what you call it, just as long as you use it! If you want to purchase only one affordable piece of equipment, get a stability ball. It can provide a great upper-body workout, a lower-body workout, a challenging abdominal workout, and can assist your stretching. How many things improve your balance and posture merely by sitting on them? Because the stability ball is an unstable surface, you have to use all of your stability muscles in your core just to balance.

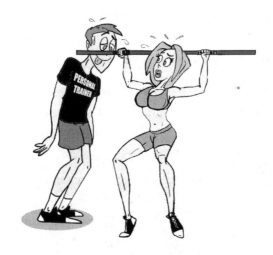

"You want to stabilize my what?!"

If you already have dumbbells, you can also use the stability ball as a weight bench.

> Beginners – two sets of 12 repetitions of each exercise
>
> Intermediate – three sets of 12 repetitions of each exercise
>
> Advanced – three sets of 15 repetitions of each exercise

Remember, you need to warm up first with 5–10 minutes of light aerobic exercise, and stretch after.

General recommended size-to-height for stability ball selection is as follows:

55 cm. ball	21 inches	4' 11" - 5' 4" tall
65 cm. ball	25 inches	5' 5" to 5' 11" tall

Stability Ball Exercises

Sitting on the Stability Ball

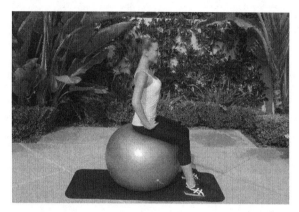

First, sit comfortably on the ball. You may want to begin with a wall or stable counter nearby, in case you lose your balance. Your feet should be wide on the floor; this makes it easier to balance. Contract your abdominals by pulling your belly button toward your spine, and begin moving your hips slightly side to side, then in small circles – in one direction, and then the other.

Ball Push-Ups

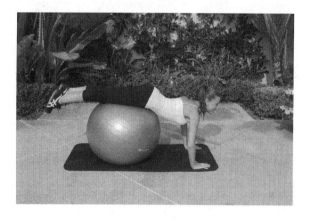

Roll forward, placing your body weight on your hands until stability ball rests under your shins. Your body should be extended in a straight line from the stability ball.

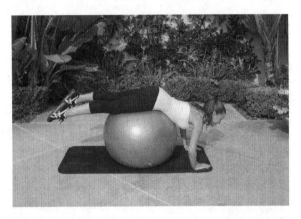

Lower your upper body toward floor, bending at the elbows to perform push-ups. Keep the abdominal muscles tight. Keep the body tight and straight from shoulders to toes.

Return to start position.

To increase difficulty, roll the ball back so only your feet are resting on it.

Abdominal Crunches

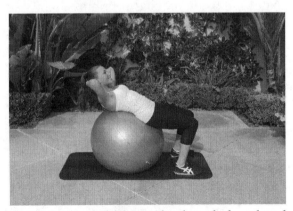

Lie with the ball resting under the mid-lower back and place hands behind the head or across the chest.

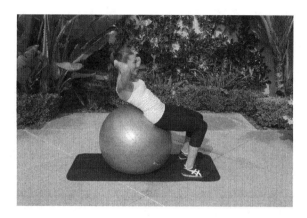

Contract your abs to lift your torso off the ball, pulling the bottom of your rib cage down toward your hips.

As you curl up, keep the ball stable.

Return to start.

Inner Thighs and Abdominals

Lie on your side with the ball between your knees or ankles, squeezing it to hold it in place.

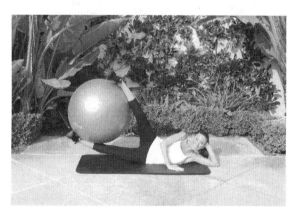

Squeeze your inner thighs and contract the waist and hip muscles to lift the ball in the air.

Lie on your back with the ball between your knees or ankles, squeezing it to hold it in place. Keep your hips stacked and abs tight to stabilize your body.

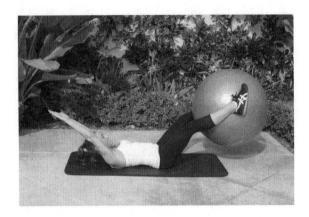

Squeeze your inner thighs and contract the waist and hip muscles to lift the ball in the air.

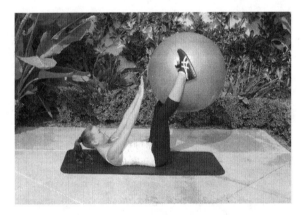

Return to start.

Back Extension

Position the ball under your hips and lower torso, with your knees straight or bent. Slowly roll down the ball.

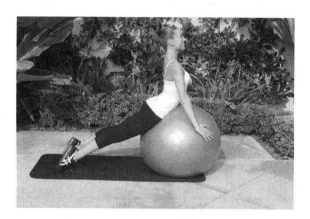

Lift your chest off the ball, bringing your shoulders up until your body is in a straight line. Make sure your body is in alignment (i.e., head, neck, shoulders, and back are in a straight line), your abs are pulled in, and you don't hyperextend the back.

Return to start.

Butt Raises
Lie on the ball with the head, neck, and shoulders supported, knees bent, and body in a "tabletop position" across the ball.

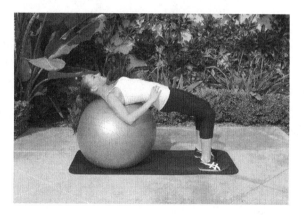

Lower the hips toward the floor without rolling on the ball.

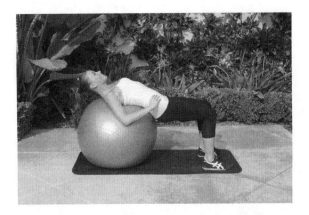

Squeeze the glutes to raise hips until body is in a straight line, like a bridge.

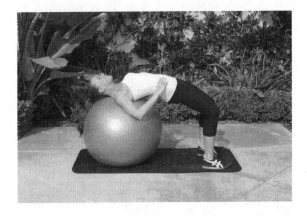

Hold weights on the hips for added intensity, and make sure you press through the heels and not the toes.

Do It Anywhere Cardio!

Don't have a treadmill or other device? You don't need one. Here are some simple cardio routines that you can do in 20–30 minutes without ANY equipment. Mix and match the moves you like best to create new routines.

Tips to Keep You Moving:
Use music that motivates you.

Keep a clock or stopwatch nearby so you can check your heart rate and keep track of the time for each "drill."

If you need to take the intensity down, march in place, but try to keep moving for the full 20–30 minutes.

WARM UP (5 minutes)
Warm up by marching in place (1 minute).

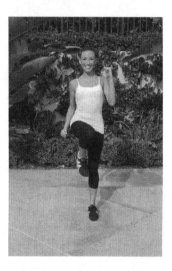

Keep marching and reach your arms overhead, alternating left and right (1 minute).

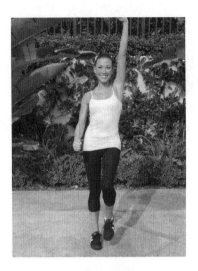

March wide, feet past the line of your hips (1 minute).

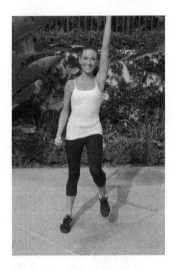

March wide, with alternating arms overhead (1 minute).

Now stretch. Bend your knees, reach up, and roll down to stretch your lower back. Round and contract your back four times. Repeat two times (1 minute).

Now, do each of the following drills for three minutes, then move on to the next.

Knees Up

March with knee raises. March right; raise your left knee toward your chest.

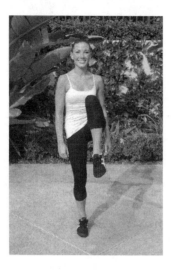

Alternate: March left, and raise your right knee to your chest.

After you feel comfortable with the knee raises, add intensity by reaching your arms up as you lift your knee and lower them as you march.

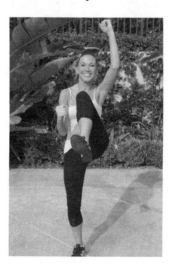

Sit Down

Imagine you are going to sit down on a chair. Lower your butt down into a squat position and stand up.

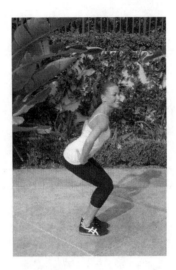

Once you feel confident doing the squat, add intensity by alternating knee raises as you stand up.

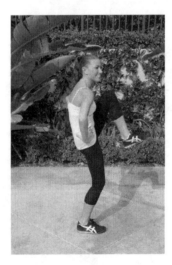

Walk It Up
March right, left tap, then march left, right tap.

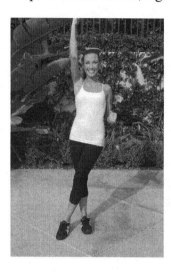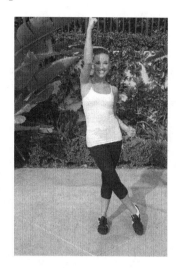

Repeat 16 times and change legs. To add intensity, lift the knee to the chest instead of tapping it on the floor.   Take the march forward and back.

"Bionic Woman" *One of my favorite butt exercises
Stand on your right foot, place your weight on your right heel, find your balance, and bring your left toe to your right heel.

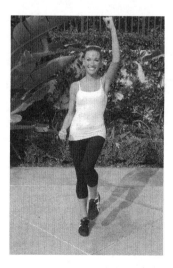

"Box It"

Alternate right and left punches. Imagine a punching bag in front of you, and keep your shoulders relaxed and hit the bag.

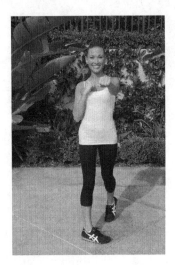

The following are 30-second drills:

"Shuffles"

With your legs in a wide stance, shuffle your feet alternating right and left.

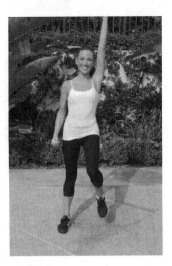

To add intensity, bring your arms up and down.

"Jack or Half Jack"
Do full jumping jacks.

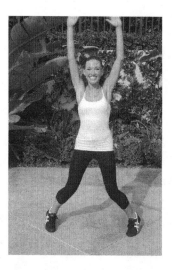

Or alternate taps side to side while bringing arms overhead.

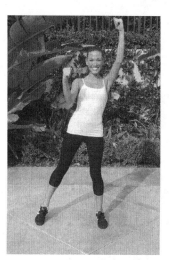 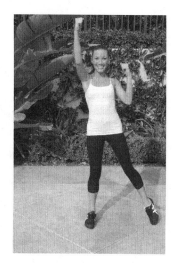

"Fancy Feet"

Alternate an imaginary jump rope, right, left double on the right. Single, single, double switch left.

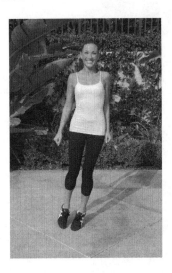 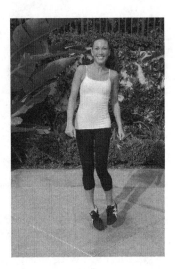

"Cancan Kicks"

Alternate kicks, keep them low and keep your abdominal muscles pulled in tight.

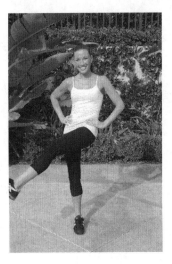

Cool Down (5 minutes)

March in place (1 minute).

March wide (1 minute).

Keep legs wide and reach arms overhead right and left as you lean side to side (1 minute).

Stretches (2 minutes)

Refer to the stretch section for flexibility options.

Putting It All Together

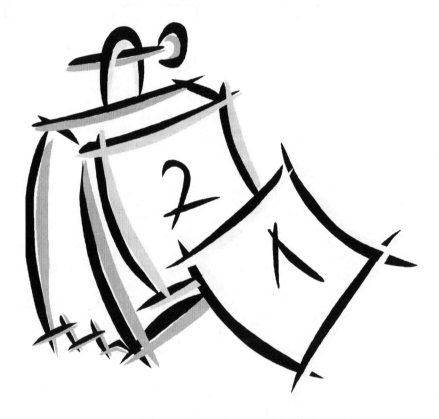

The 21-Day Dump Your Trainer Diet & Fitness Program

Get Ready to Change How You Look and Feel in Just 21 Days.

The 21-Day Dump Your Trainer Diet & Fitness Program is the time to challenge yourself and create a new you. This is the most restrictive part of the program. You will be following this meal and exercise plan for 21 days. This is the time to break unwanted "food addictions" and retrain your body and mind to crave healthy foods.

*Warning: This intensive program is not advisable for anyone suffering from a medical condition, or for pregnant or lactating women. Seek the advice of your doctor before beginning any diet program.

Why 21 Days?
Because 21 days of dedicated thought and consistent action, toward the change you want, will create a desired habit while replacing an unwanted behavior.

Dr. Maxwell Maltz (1899–1976) wrote the bestseller *Psycho-Cybernetics*. Originally a plastic surgeon, Maltz noticed that it took 21 days for amputees to cease feeling phantom sensations in the amputated limb. From further observations, he found it took 21 days to create a new habit.

Brain circuits take engrams (memory traces), and produce neuro-connections and neuro-pathways only if they are bombarded for 21 days in a row. This means that our brain does not accept "new" data for a change of habit unless it is repeated each day for 21 days, without missing a day.

The new habit needs to take the place of a previously entrenched old one. Old habits are not so easily overruled. The new habit will need to be supported and encouraged to have any chance of survival.

21-Day Transformation Steps

Make the decision.

See It
Create the image of your goal in your mind. Take a few minutes each day to visualize your goal. See yourself overflowing with health and energy. You may want to use a picture of yourself at your ideal weight, a picture from a magazine, the number you want to see on the scale, or the clothing size you want to wear.

Say It
Choose the habit you most want to focus on for the next 21 days. Repeat an auto-suggestion phrase 20 times when you wake up and 20 times before you go to sleep.

Example: Habit – Eating late at night.

"I only eat before seven p.m.; I am in control of when I eat; I no longer eat after seven p.m."

Write It
Writing down your goal is a commitment to achieve it. Taking the time to focus, visualize, and write down your specific goal creates momentum that will fuel your actions. Write your goal as if it has already been achieved: I am so happy now that

_____.

Success Strategies

In order for you to maximize your weight loss and fitness program, it's highly recommended that you follow these suggestions:

Exercise: This program should be integrated with The 21-Day Dump Your Trainer Fitness Program.

Water: Please remember to drink 8–10 glasses of filtered water each day.

Alcohol: If at all possible, avoid alcohol. Cutting out alcohol, especially during the first 21 days, can add an additional two to three pounds of weight loss per week and greatly increase your energy level.

Stop Eating At Least Three Hours Before Going To Sleep: By imposing an eating cut-off time of three (or more) hours before bed, we automatically slash our caloric intake, commonly cutting 500–1000 calories per day, which can add up to an additional two pounds of additional weight loss per week.

Combine these two, and you'll be looking at an additional five pounds of weight loss per week.

The best way to get rid of an unwanted habit is to replace it with a good habit for 21 consecutive days.

Food List

Make sure to stock up on the following items:

Vegetables: Asparagus, Bell Pepper, Bok Choy, Broccoli, Brussels Sprouts, Cabbage, Cauliflower, Celery, Chard, Collard Greens, Cucumber, Eggplant, Kale, Mushrooms, Onion, Peppers, Radishes, Spinach, Sprouts, String Beans, Yellow Squash, Zucchini

Lettuce: Romaine, endive and similar leafy greens, iceberg

Toppings/Mixers: Mustard, salsa, low-calorie flavored/unflavored water for mixing your smoothies, nonfat whey or soy protein powder

Meats: Chicken breast, fish, turkey, lean steak, lean lamb, pork tenderloin, extra-lean turkey slices, extra-lean chicken slices, and eggs

Meat Substitutes: BOCA burgers or other soy burgers with less than four grams of fat per serving, tofu, tempeh, low-fat soy cheese, low-fat soy yogurt, eggs, soybeans

Fruits: Blueberries, Strawberries, Blackberries, Boysenberries, Raspberries, Apples, Pears, Nectarines, Melon, Oranges, Peaches, Grapefruit, Kiwi, Plums, Tangerines

Note: During the first 7–21 days, any between-meal snacks should preferably be boiled egg whites or 99% fat-free turkey breast, ham, or chicken slices and topped with mustard, if desired. Fruit can be eaten sparingly during the first 7–21 days, after which it can be added more liberally.

Snack Options

Each snack should be between 170–200 calories:

> Popcorn and a no-oil microwave popper (Note: you can pick one up at Target)
> Uncooked (soft) whole wheat or fat-free tortillas
> 1 serving fruit
> 1 serving string cheese with small fruit
> 1 oz. roast turkey wrapped round celery or carrot sticks
> 3 oz. fresh tuna with 2 cups of lettuce
> 1 cup veggies with 2 Tbsp. nonfat dressing
> 2 cups salad with 2 Tbsp. nonfat dressing

Whey protein shake
1/2 cup nonfat cottage cheese with small fruit

General Notes

If you do the aerobic exercise program in the morning as recommended, you may not be hungry for a fair part of the morning. If you're at the office or out on the road, you'll likely have a mid-morning meal instead of breakfast. Prepare for this with a selection of pre-pared protein smoothies.

Preparing for the 21-Day Dump Your Trainer Diet & Fitness Program

Strategic Plan

"People with goals succeed because they know where they are going." – Earl Nightingale

During the next 21 days, you'll transform your old behaviors/habits and create new ones to support your goals. Each day, for 21 consecutive days, you will be using the 21-Day Dump Your Trainer Program to establish your new healthy lifestyle goals.

The first step in making a real commitment is your belief in yourself; "I am doing this," instead of "I'm going to try to do it." The language you use is just as important as your physical action. Create an inner and outer dialogue that is focused on the results you want. Know that you have the power to change your behavior and create the outcome you desire.

Take a few minutes to answer the following questions, writing down the first three answers that come to mind:

Why do you want to change your body?

1.

2.

3.

What is preventing you from achieving your goal?

1.

2.

3.

You Can Do It!

Start with a Personal Success Contract. Read the following contract, which you'll be making with yourself and resolve to honor it from now on. Energize your goal today by signing your contract.

Personal Success Contract

I, _____ , commit to starting my fitness program today, _____.

I commit to using the Dump Your Trainer – Change Your Life Workout Program consistently and following the Dump Your Trainer – Dump the Weight healthful eating program that will help me attain my fitness and health goals.

I will only fuel my body with the most nutritious foods possible.

I will be kind to myself and appreciate all that my body does for me.

I will strive to challenge my body and my mind.

I will acknowledge and reward myself for my achievements along the way.

_____

Signature

Day One

"A goal is nothing more than a dream with a deadline."

Action Step

Energize your goal today by signing your Success Contract and beginning The 21-Day Dump Your Trainer Diet & Fitness Plan.

Morning weigh in (It all begins here!)

Morning walk/jog/bike or Ashley's "Burn 'N Firm" – Total Fitness DVD

Breakfast or Mid-morning Meal
Coffee/tea/

Blended smoothie with 1–2 scoops protein powder

OR:

6–10 hardboiled egg whites

6 oz. vegetable juice

Lunch
Grilled skinless chicken breast

Steamed broccoli and cauliflower

Iced tea/natural low calorie soda

Afternoon Snack
Protein smoothie

Evening exercise

Aerobics dance class/elliptical trainer/treadmill/bike; plus 20 minutes of toning

Evening weigh in

Dinner

    Grilled salmon

    Steamed vegetables

    Caffeine-free soda/iced tea/water

Evening Snack – optional

    Microwave oil-free popcorn

    Raw vegetables (celery sticks, baby carrots, broccoli, etc.) with fat-free dressing dip, if desired

Day Two

"You must first see a thing in your mind before you can do it." – Alex Morison

Action Step

Take a few minutes today and visualize the body you want. Create the image in rich detail, focusing on the positive changes that are occurring now. You may want to use real pictures, as well – a favorite prior photo of yourself, a body you admire that will remind you of your goal.

Take action by eating a healthy breakfast. People who regularly skip breakfast are four times as likely to be obese than those who eat breakfast. Breakfast eaters consume less fat during the day and have lower cholesterol levels than those who don't.

NOTE: If you follow the Dump Your Trainer morning exercise program and don't feel hungry for a while afterward, prepare for this with a pre-made mid-morning breakfast or nutritious smoothie. Don't wait until lunch to eat – your resistance to "pigging out" will be insurmountable.

Morning weigh in

Morning walk/jog/bike or "Burn 'N Firm" – Total Fitness DVD

Breakfast or Mid-morning Meal

Coffee/tea/or personal choice

Blended smoothie with 1–2 scoops protein powder

OR:

Egg white omelet with salsa

6 oz. vegetable juice

Lunch

    Roasted skinless turkey breast

    Mixed salad with fat-free dressing, if needed or steamed vegetables

    Iced tea/natural low calorie soda

Afternoon Snack

    Protein smoothie

Evening exercise

Aerobics dance class/elliptical trainer/treadmill/bike; plus 20 minutes of toning

Evening weigh in

Dinner

    Grilled halibut

    Steamed vegetables

    Caffeine-free soda/iced tea/water

Evening Snack – optional

    Baked/toasted tortilla and salsa

    Cherry tomatoes and cucumber slices with fat-free dressing dip, if desired

Day Three

Action Step

Decide what you want. Decide what you are willing to exchange for it.

Step One

> Each day, take a look at one behavior you want to change.

Step Two

> Write a list of the reasons why you want to change.

Step Three

Write one action you will take NOW to change that behavior and how you will feel when you are free from the behavior.

EXAMPLE

Step One

> Quit snacking when I watch TV.

Step Two

> Eating mindlessly makes me feel bad – I could be doing other things – I don't feel productive – it wastes my time.

Step Three

> I will not eat when I watch TV.

> I feel proud of myself!

The average American spends 30–40 hours per week watching TV – a completely sedentary activity. If you are watching TV, make commercial breaks a mini workout – stretch, march in place, do a quick set of squats, or even jumping jacks.

Morning weigh in

Morning walk/jog/bike or Ashley's "Burn 'N Firm" – Total Fitness DVD

Breakfast or Mid-morning Meal

Coffee/tea/or personal choice

Blended smoothie with 1–2 scoops protein powder

OR:

Scrambled egg whites with peppers and onions

6 oz. vegetable juice

Lunch

Lean steak

Steamed broccoli and cauliflower

Iced tea/natural low calorie soda

Afternoon Snack

Protein smoothie

Evening exercise

Aerobics dance class/elliptical trainer/treadmill/bike; plus 20 minutes of toning

Evening weigh in

Dinner

Grilled haddock

Steamed cauliflower

Caffeine-free soda/iced tea/water

Evening Snack – optional

Microwave oil-free popcorn

Raw vegetables (celery sticks, baby carrots, broccoli, etc.) with fat-free dressing dip, if desired

Day Four

"Your focus is everything." – William James

Action Step

Today, focus on all the positive actions you are taking to attain your healthy ideal body.

Step One

> Close your eyes and create a feeling of certainty that you will achieve your goal.

Step Two

> Take a deep breath. As you exhale, release any doubt, fear, or limiting beliefs that may have blocked you from reaching your goal in the past.

Step Three

> Open your eyes with a feeling of certainty that your goal will be achieved.

Repeat this process each morning and evening.

Morning weigh in

Morning walk/jog/bike or Ashley's "Burn 'N Firm" – Total Fitness DVD

Breakfast or Mid-morning Meal

> Coffee/tea/or personal choice

> Blended smoothie with 1–2 scoops protein powder

OR:

Egg white cheese omelet with fat-free cheese and tomatoes

6 oz. vegetable juice

Lunch

Lean hamburger with mustard, lettuce, tomato, and onion, without the bun

Iced tea/natural low calorie soda

Afternoon Snack

Protein smoothie

Evening exercise

Aerobics dance class/elliptical trainer/treadmill/bike; plus 20 minutes of toning

Evening weigh in

Dinner

Baked skinless chicken breast

Steamed vegetables

Caffeine-free soda/iced tea/water

Evening Snack – optional

Baked/toasted tortilla and salsa

Day Five

"We are what we think about all day long." – Ralph Waldo Emerson

Your thoughts are in your control, and they can be very powerful. Positive thoughts can motivate healthy behaviors, such as eating right and being active. It's simple, really. If you believe you can take 10,000 steps a day, you will be more likely to take an extra walk to meet your goal.

But the reverse is also true. Your thoughts can be defeating. "I've already messed up on my meal plan, so it doesn't matter if I eat a second piece of cake."

Negative thoughts and negative self-talk may sabotage your good intentions. Positive thinking can help you achieve and maintain healthy behaviors.

Studies have measured the success of positive thinkers and found that those who think they can lose weight, or increase their physical activity, do! These people are more successful than people with less faith in themselves. The confidence you have in performing a certain behavior is called self-efficacy, and self-efficacy is a key in successful behavior change.

Action Step

Want Results?
Can-Do!

Many professional athletes get top sports training and coaching in positive thinking to help them achieve their goals. And it works! The same can apply for you and me. A "can-do" attitude may be just what it takes to jumpstart a healthier lifestyle. Best of all, your attitude is something you can control.

You have the choice to have a positive outlook. Chances are, when you choose to think positively, you'll feel better about yourself and be able to perform better in whatever you do.

Stay On Track

There will be days when you don't feel like working out, slip from eating right, or lose your temper. Small setbacks are part of life. Learn from your past successes and failures.

Don't dwell on the past. Learn and move on, so next time you'll make healthier choices toward positive change.

How to Stay Positive

Positive thinkers admit when they feel frustrated or depressed. They don't ignore it. But they also don't blame themselves. Instead, they try to understand the negative thoughts and feelings, and counter them with more positive ones.

So, how do you stay positive, maintain momentum, and sustain healthy behaviors?

1. Take a minute to give yourself an ego boost. Repeat some motivational words out loud or to yourself.

2. Avoid negative talk, such as "I'm not good at this." It's dangerous for your well-being and healthy goals. Try to avoid the negative inner voice.

3. Remind yourself that you deserve happiness and are making positive changes.

Get support. Tell your friends and family about your healthy habits. It helps to have a supportive network. But remember, don't become reliant on anyone else to achieve your goals.

Reward yourself. Give yourself a pat on the back for all your healthy efforts. Get a massage, go to a show, or enjoy a new DVD or CD.

Have a plan. Making a plan to exercise or eat healthy lunches can mean the difference between sticking with your goals or falling off track. If you've planned for an activity, you are likely to stick with it. Take it day by day or week by week.

The process of writing down your personal action plan is a good way to keep you honest, watch your progress, or notice your pitfalls.

Think positive thoughts while you work out. Use thoughts like "The world looks good. I'm glad I'm training today. I feel great." Avoid thoughts like "I'm tired. I'm not improving." Remember that your training session is probably the only time you'll have all day that's just for you. You want it to be as pleasant, positive, and productive as possible.

Morning weigh in

Morning walk/jog/bike or Ashley's "Burn 'N Firm" – Total Fitness DVD

Breakfast or Mid-morning Meal

Coffee/tea/or personal choice

Blended smoothie with 1–2 scoops protein powder

OR:

6–10 hardboiled egg whites

6 oz. vegetable juice

Lunch

Two-cheese (fat-free) skinless chicken breast tacos with salsa

Iced tea/natural low calorie soda

Afternoon Snack

Protein smoothie

Evening exercise

Aerobics dance class/elliptical trainer/treadmill/bike; plus 20 minutes of toning

Evening weigh in

Dinner

Skinless Cornish hen

Mixed salad with fat-free dressing, if needed

Caffeine-free soda/tea/water

Evening Snack – optional

Microwave oil-free popcorn

Cherry tomatoes and cucumber slices with fat-free dressing dip, if desired

Day Six

"Every day I count wasted in which there has been no dancing." – Friederich Nietzsche

Action Step

Fitness has many forms. Add a physical activity that you enjoy – hiking, biking, dancing, swimming, yoga, or a walk in a beautiful setting. Fully immerse yourself in it and feel the rhythm of it. Look for new opportunities to move more every day. Our bodies are gifts. The fitter we become, the more we can fully experience the joy of movement each day.

Morning weigh in

Morning walk/jog/bike or Ashley's "Burn 'N Firm" – Total Fitness DVD

Breakfast or Mid-morning Meal
>   Coffee/tea/or personal choice
>
>   Blended smoothie with 1–2 scoops protein powder
>
>   **OR:**
>
>   6–10 hardboiled egg whites
>
>   6 oz. vegetable juice

Lunch
>   Grilled skinless chicken breast
>
>   Steamed green beans and carrots
>
>   Iced tea/natural low calorie soda

Afternoon Snack
>   Protein smoothie

Evening exercise

Aerobics dance class/elliptical trainer/treadmill/bike; plus 20 minutes of toning

Evening weigh in

Dinner

Broiled cod

Steamed vegetables

Caffeine-free soda/iced tea/water

Evening Snack – optional

Baked/toasted tortilla and salsa

Day Seven

"Discipline means choices. Every time you say yes to a goal or objective you say no to many more." – Sybil Stanton

Action Step

You can always make a healthy choice.

Commit to make the best health choices possible – even at the drive-through window.

Morning weigh in

Morning walk/jog/bike or Ashley's "Burn 'N Firm" – Total Fitness DVD

Breakfast or Mid-morning Meal

> Coffee/tea/or personal choice

> Blended smoothie with 1–2 scoops protein powder

> **OR:**

> 2 low-fat soft tacos with 4 (2+2) hardboiled eggs whites with fat-free cheese and salsa. Microwave taco sized tostadas and cheese then add chopped egg whites and warm salsa.

> 6 oz. vegetable juice

Lunch

> Two grilled skinless chicken breasts

> Iced tea/natural low calorie soda

Afternoon Snack

> Protein smoothie

Evening exercise

Aerobics dance class/elliptical trainer/treadmill/bike; plus 20 minutes of toning

Evening weigh in

Dinner

Skinless Cornish hen

Mixed salad with fat-free dressing, if needed

Caffeine-free soda/tea/water

Evening Snack – optional

Rolled turkey slices with/without mustard

Raw vegetables (celery sticks, baby carrots, broccoli, etc.) with fat-free dressing dip, if desired

Day Eight

"Success is the sum of small efforts, repeated day in and day out."– Robert Collier

Action Step

Get moving! Everything counts when it comes to physical activity.

Sixty minutes of The Dump Your Trainer workout will burn approximately 400–500 calories.

Walking – 10 minutes of brisk walking will burn approximately 100 calories.

Swimming – 10 minutes of swimming laps.

Biking – 40 minutes.

Stairs – climbing stairs for 20 minutes will burn approximately 100 calories.

Housework – 20 minutes will burn approximately 100 calories.

Gardening – 20 minutes will burn approximately 100 calories.

All of these "small efforts" can really make a difference at the end of the month. If you add one per day, along with three Dump Your Trainer aerobic sessions, that's approximately 4,200 calories burned per month.

Check out http://www.healthstatus.com to find out how many calories you burn doing other activities.

Morning weigh in

Morning walk/jog/bike or Ashley's "Burn 'N Firm" – Total Fitness DVD

Breakfast or mid-morning meal.
Whey protein shake (TBA brand) mixed with 5 oz. nonfat milk, soy milk, or half milk and half water; mix in a blender with ice

OR:

Egg white omelet

> 6 egg whites, lightly beaten
>
> 1 tsp. olive oil
>
> 1/2 cup chopped red pepper
>
> 1/2 cup diced zucchini
>
> 1 small tomato
>
> 3 sprigs fresh basil (or dry)
>
> 1 clove chopped garlic
>
> NO SALT
>
> Put olive oil in pan; add garlic, veggies, and basil. Cook over medium heat, stirring frequently. Add egg whites and scramble until cooked.

Lunch

Tuna Salad

6 oz. water-packed tuna, drained

2 slices of tomato

1 cup romaine (or baby mixed greens)

1 cup cucumber and celery

Place salad ingredients in a bowl.

2 Tbsp. Non/low fat, low sugar dressing

OR:

4 oz. skinless chicken breast, grilled, with no oil

1 cup of vegetables

Afternoon Snack
>   Protein smoothie

Evening exercise

Aerobics dance class/elliptical trainer/treadmill/bike; plus 20 minutes of toning

Evening weigh in

Dinner
>   Tofu-Vegetable Stir-Fry

>>   1 oz. extra firm tofu, cubed

>>   1 cup vegetables (bell peppers, mushrooms, onion, broccoli)

>>   1 garlic clove

>>   1/4 Tbsp. red pepper flakes

>>   Spray wok or nonstick skillet with nonfat cooking spray. Sauté red pepper flakes on medium-high heat; add garlic, onion, and vegetables. Cook for 2–3 minutes, add tofu and stir-fry until heated through.

>   **OR:**

>   4 oz. protein from list

>   1 cup vegetables

Evening Snack – optional
>   Microwave oil-free popcorn

>   Cherry tomatoes and cucumber slices with fat-free dressing dip, if desired

Day Nine

"In truth the only difference between those who have failed and those who have succeeded lies in the difference of their habits." – Og Mandino

Action Step

Take Action by Eliminating the "Try."

Often, we talk to ourselves and others using the word "try" rather than "will." Have you ever heard yourself saying "I'll try to eat healthy," or "I'll try to work out," or "I'll try to drink more water"? Watch how you talk to yourself and others about your fitness goals and habits. Use the words "I will" and "I am," and follow up with actions that align affirmative words with positive behavior. These habits will become your routine and success will breed more success.

Step One

Stay On Track

Keep with the plan, focus on your goal.

Step Two

Stay Positive

1. Take a minute to give yourself an ego boost. Repeat some motivational words out loud or to yourself.

2. Avoid negative talk, such as "I'm not good at this" or "I can't do it."

3. Remind yourself that you deserve happiness and you ARE making positive changes.

Step Three

Get support. Tell your friends and family about your healthy habits!

Morning weigh in

Morning walk/jog/bike or Ashley's "Burn 'N Firm" – Total Fitness DVD

Breakfast or Mid-morning Meal

    1 cup oatmeal

    2 slices turkey bacon or 2 soy sausage links

OR:

Whey protein shake (see Day Eight)

Lunch

    Bun-free burger

        1 extra lean patty

        2 oz. low-fat cheese

        4 leaves green lettuce

        1 Tbsp. mustard

        Cook patty with cheese on top, place on lettuce.

OR:

Spinach salad

        1 cup fresh spinach

        1 hardboiled egg

        3 oz. sliced grilled chicken breast

        1 cup shredded vegetables

        1/2 cup sliced mushrooms

    2 Tbsp. low-fat dressing

Afternoon Snack

    Protein smoothie

Evening exercise

Aerobics dance class/elliptical trainer/treadmill/bike; plus 20 minutes of toning

Evening weigh in

Dinner

Beef Tenderloin and Mashed Cauliflower

4 oz. grilled beef tenderloin

1 cup mixed salad greens

2 Tbsp. low-cal dressing

1 medium head cauliflower, cut into florets

1 cup purified water

2 garlic cloves, minced

1 tsp. fresh chives, chopped

1/2 tsp. onion powder

1/2 tsp. fresh parsley, chopped

1 Tbsp. chicken broth

In a medium pot, place cauliflower with water and bring to a quick boil. Lower heat to simmer and cover. Cook for an additional 12 minutes or until soft. Drain; transfer cauliflower to a bowl and mash. Blend in garlic, chives, onion powder, parsley, and broth with the mashed cauliflower. Serve hot.

OR:

4 oz. protein from option list

1 cup vegetables

Evening Snack – optional

Baked/toasted tortilla and salsa

Day Ten

"If you want your future to be different than your past study your past." –
Baruch Spinoza

Action Step

Step One

> Write down three negative beliefs that have kept you from achieving your health/fitness goals.

Step Two

> Write down three actions you are taking NOW to eliminate these limiting thoughts.

Step Three

> Write down three ways your life will improve after you are free of the negative beliefs.

Move forward from this day empowered with a new understanding of who you are becoming, knowing you are moving closer and closer to your fitness goals!

Example:

Step One

> 1) I can't change my body.
>
> 2) I don't like to exercise.
>
> 3) I like to eat junk food.

Step Two

> 1) I'm losing weight.
>
> 2) I enjoy how strong I feel when I exercise.

3) I am in control of everything I eat.

Step Three

1) I will feel and look wonderful!

2) I will feel strong and healthy, and excited to take on new challenges.

3) I will be proud that I take care of my body and appreciate my great health.

Morning weigh in

Morning walk/jog/bike or Ashley's "Burn 'N Firm" – Total Fitness DVD

Breakfast or Mid-morning Meal

Whey protein shake (see Day Eight)

OR:

Omelet with Cheese

6 egg whites

2 Tbsp. red and/or green bell pepper

1 Tbsp. scallions

2 Tbsp. reduced fat cheese

Spray nonstick cooking pan with cooking spray. Add pepper and scallions. Pour in egg whites. Add cheese. Fold.

Lunch

3 oz. slices of turkey, chicken, or tofu

4 leaves of lettuce

1/2 bell pepper, cut into strips

1 tsp. reduced fat mayo, mustard, or 1 Tbsp. reduced fat salad dressing

Place meat on lettuce, spread with mayo, and roll it up.

OR:

Grilled or Baked Chicken Salad

> 3 oz. Grilled or baked chicken
>
> 2 cup lettuce
>
> 1/2 cup vegetables
>
> 2 Tbsp. low-cal dressing

Afternoon Snack
Protein smoothie

Evening exercise

Aerobics dance class/elliptical trainer/treadmill/bike; plus 20 minutes of toning

Evening weigh in

Dinner
Lemon Chicken Breast

> 1 skinless boneless chicken thigh
>
> Lemon juice
>
> 1 shallot
>
> 1/2 Tbsp. capers
>
> 1 Tbsp. Dijon mustard
>
> 1 cup steamed vegetables
>
> Place the chicken in a shallow roasting pan and cover with the sauce. Broil for 12–15 minutes until chicken is fully cooked.

OR:

4 oz. protein from option list

1 cup vegetables

Evening Snack – optional

Microwave oil-free popcorn

Raw vegetables (celery sticks, baby carrots, broccoli, etc.) with fat-free dressing dip, if desired

Day Eleven

"Mind, body and spirit act in concert to determine health and well being." –
Dr. Carl Thoresen

Action Step

Focus on your well-being. Health is a state of complete physical, mental, and social well-being, and not merely the absence of disease or infirmity.

Keeping track of your waist measurement is an easy way to measure the progress that you are making. The recommended waist measurement for women is 32" or less, and the healthy waist measurement for a man is 35" or less.

Morning weigh in

Morning walk/jog/bike or Ashley's "Burn 'N Firm" – Total Fitness DVD

Breakfast or Mid-morning Meal
Salmon Scramble

> 2 eggs or 6 egg whites

> 1 oz. smoked salmon, cut in thin strips

> 1 Tbsp. chives or other herbs, to taste

> Heat nonfat cooking spray in nonstick pan over medium heat for 1 minute. Add eggs, salmon, and herbs.

OR:

1 cup oatmeal

2 slices turkey bacon or 2 soy sausage links

Lunch
Grilled Hamburger Patty on Lettuce

1 extra lean hamburger patty

2 cups lettuce

2 Tbsp. nonfat dressing

1 cup vegetables

OR:

Tofu Salad

1/2 cup firm tofu, cubed

2 cups mixed green salad

1/2 vegetables

1 tsp. sesame seeds

2 Tbsp. nonfat dressing

Afternoon Snack

Protein smoothie

Evening exercise

Aerobics dance class/elliptical trainer/treadmill/bike; plus 20 minutes of toning

Evening weigh in

Dinner

Whey protein shake (see Day Eight)

OR:

4 oz. protein from option list

1 cup vegetables

Evening Snack – optional

Rolled turkey slices with/without mustard

Cherry tomatoes and cucumber slices with fat-free dressing dip, if desired

Day Twelve

"Many of life's failures are people who did not realize how close they were to success when they gave up." – Thomas Edison

Action Step

Use your positive progress to push forward.

1. Be sure to celebrate your accomplishments during your program. Be proud of yourself for all your hard work, for better food choices, and even for drinking that extra sip of water.

2. Refuse to put down or belittle yourself. Don't dwell on the things you didn't do perfectly this week. Choose to move forward instead of remaining stuck in the past.

3. Reward yourself and take time to enjoy one of your favorite activities – reading a good book, taking a hot bath, going to a movie, taking a nap, going out with family and friends, getting a manicure, a pedicure, a massage, or anything that satisfies your soul.

Morning weigh in

Morning walk/jog/bike or Ashley's "Burn 'N Firm" – Total Fitness DVD

Breakfast or Mid-morning Meal
Egg white omelet (see Day Eight)

OR:

Whey protein shake (see Day Eight)

Lunch
Ham or Turkey Sandwich

1 whole wheat pita

3 oz. lean ham or turkey

Mustard

1 Tbsp. reduced fat mayo

3 leaves romaine lettuce

OR:

Better BOCABurger

BOCA or veggie burger

1 whole wheat toasted bun

1 Tbsp. olive oil

2 slices of tomato

3 leaves of lettuce

1 slice red onion

Afternoon Snack

Protein smoothie

Evening exercise

Aerobics dance class/elliptical trainer/treadmill/bike; plus 20 minutes of toning

Evening weigh in

Dinner

Salmon & Vegetables

1 salmon fillet, grilled with nonfat cooking spray for 8 –10 minutes

1 cup steamed vegetables

OR:

4 oz. protein from option list

1 cup vegetables

Evening Snack – optional
Baked/toasted tortilla and salsa

Day Thirteen

"Appreciation can make a day, even change a life. Your willingness to put it into words is all that is necessary." – Margaret Cousins

Action Step

Start a Gratitude Journal

Sarah Breathnach describes the benefits of keeping a Gratitude Journal in her book, *Simple Abundance*. She states that a Gratitude Journal can "change the quality of your life beyond belief."

Before you go to sleep, record five things you are grateful for. Your outlook on life will change as you continue to keep your gratitude journal, because you will be looking for the things you are thankful for each day and recording them later in your journal. This process produces positive results in all areas of one's life, including the area of health and fitness.

When recording what you are grateful for, be conscious of noting feelings of gratitude that are affecting your physical body and health.

Examples could be "I am grateful for drinking 10 glasses of water today to cleanse my body, I am grateful for how strong I feel, I am grateful for the long walk/run I took today, I am grateful for the people who support my health, I am grateful for making good food choices at the restaurant today, or simply I am grateful for my body."

Morning weigh in

Morning walk/jog/bike or Ashley's "Burn 'N Firm" – Total Fitness DVD

Breakfast or Mid-morning Meal

    1 cup oatmeal

    2 slices turkey bacon or 2 soy sausage links

OR:

Whey protein shake (see Day Eight)

Lunch

Tuna Salad

> 6 oz. water-packed tuna, drained

> 2 slices of tomato

> 1 cup romaine (or baby mixed greens)

> 1 cup cucumber and celery

> Place salad ingredients in a bowl. Add 1/2 tsp. relish; mix tuna, mayo, and celery.

> 2 tbsp. low fat dressing

OR:

Roll Ups

> 3 oz. sliced turkey, ham, chicken, or tofu

> 4 leaves of lettuce

> 1/2 bell pepper, cut into strips

> 1 tsp. reduced fat mayo, mustard, or 1 Tbsp. reduced fat salad dressing

> Place meat on lettuce, spread with mayo, and roll it up.

Afternoon Snack

Protein smoothie

Evening exercise

Aerobics dance class/elliptical trainer/treadmill/bike; plus 20 minutes of toning

Evening weigh in

Dinner

Steak & Broccoli

4–6 oz. lean filet or sirloin steak

1 tsp. olive oil

Brush the steak with the oil on sides, then grill or barbecue to taste.

1 cup steamed broccoli

OR:

4 oz. protein from option list

1 cup vegetables

Evening Snack – optional

Rolled turkey slices with/without mustard

Raw vegetables (celery sticks, baby carrots, broccoli, etc.) with fat-free dressing dip, if desired

Day Fourteen

"First we form habits, then they form us. Conquer your bad habits, or they'll eventually conquer you." – Ancient Proverb

Action Step

Recognize your progress and recommit. Acknowledge all of the changes you've made along the way. Write down all the things that have improved for you. Do you have more energy? Have you lost pounds and inches? Are you eating healthier? Has the way you look at your health changed? Large or small, all improvements matter.

Evaluate your progress. Only you know if you can "raise the bar" and push yourself more to achieve the goals you have set for yourself. As you progress through your program, look at your goals again and recommit yourself to positive change. You are on the right path! Remind yourself of where you are going and what it takes to get there!

Morning weigh in

Morning walk/jog/bike or Ashley's "Burn 'N Firm" – Total Fitness DVD

Breakfast or Mid-morning Meal
>Coffee/tea/or personal choice

>Egg white omelet (see Day Eight)

>OR:

>Whey protein shake (see Day Eight)

Lunch
>Turkey Sandwich

>>1 whole wheat pita

>>3 oz. lean turkey

>>Mustard

1 Tbsp. reduced fat mayo

3 leaves of romaine

OR:

Tofu Salad

1/2 cup firm tofu, cubed

2 cups mixed green salad

1/2 vegetables

1 tsp. sesame seeds

2 Tbsp. nonfat dressing

Afternoon Snack

Protein smoothie

Evening exercise

Aerobics dance class/elliptical trainer/treadmill/bike; plus 20 minutes of toning

Evening weigh in

Dinner

Chicken Breast and Vegetables

4 oz. skinless boneless chicken breast baked with seasoning

1 cup green beans or other vegetable

OR:

4 oz. protein from option list

1 cup vegetables

Evening Snack – optional

Microwave oil-free popcorn

Cherry tomatoes and cucumber slices with fat-free dressing dip, if desired

Day Fifteen

"While we may not be able to control all that happens to us, we can control what happens inside us." – Ben Franklin

Action Step

Practice eating mindfully. Consider the following suggestions:

Breathe deeply and relax before you eat.

Eat sitting down.

Eat without TV, newspaper, or computer.

Chew your food 30–50 times per bite.

Eating while multitasking, driving, working through lunch, or watching TV often leads us to eat more than we realize. On the other hand, eating "mindfully," savoring every mouthful, enhances the experience of eating and keeps us aware of how much we take in. Stephanie Vangsness, R.D., L.D.N., C.N.S.D., author of the article "Mindful Eating," www.intelihealth.com/IH/ihtIH/EMIHC267/35320/35327/418325.html describes this behavior as follows: "…66% of Americans report regularly eating dinner in front of the television. With obesity at epidemic proportions, it is essential that we look at not just what we eat, but how we eat."

"Scientists are beginning to evaluate and better understand the complex role of the mind-body connection in eating behavior. It turns out that when our mind is tuned out during mealtime, the digestive process may be 30% to 40% less effective. This can contribute to digestive distress, such as gas, bloating and bowel irregularities. Gas and bloating aside, overeating and obesity are perhaps the most significant health problems caused, at least in part, by mindless eating."

"The mind-body connection plays a pivotal role in our ability to accurately assess hunger and fullness. While the precise mechanisms of hunger and fullness are not completely understood, we do know that the brain and central nervous system receive signals from the body when food is desired or needed. These signals can be caused by many triggers, including psychological states such as our mood."

"Once eating is under way, the brain has a key role to send out a signal when fullness is approaching. If the mind is 'multi-tasking' during eating, critical signals that regulate food intake may not be received by the brain. If the brain does not receive certain messages that occur during eating, such as sensation of taste and satisfaction, it may fail to register the event as 'eating.' This scenario can lead to the brain's continuing to send out additional signals of hunger, increasing the risk of overeating."

Morning weigh in

Morning walk/jog/bike or Ashley's "Burn 'N Firm" – Total Fitness DVD

Breakfast or Mid-morning Meal

Coffee/tea/or personal choice

Blended smoothie with 1–2 scoops protein powder

OR:

1 cup oatmeal

1/2 cup skim milk or soy milk

2 slices turkey bacon or 2 soy sausage links

1 fruit

Lunch

Grilled skinless chicken breast

Steamed broccoli and cauliflower

Iced tea/natural low calorie soda

Afternoon Snack

Protein smoothie

Evening exercise

Aerobics dance class/elliptical trainer/treadmill/bike; plus 20 minutes of toning

Evening weigh in

Dinner

>Grilled salmon

>Steamed vegetables

>Caffeine-free soda/iced tea/water

Evening Snack – optional

>Microwave oil-free popcorn

>Raw vegetables (celery sticks, baby carrots, broccoli, etc.) with fat-free dressing dip, if desired

Day Sixteen

"Virtually nothing on earth can stop a person with a positive attitude who has their goal clearly in sight." – Denis Waitley

Action Step

Positive thinking + Positive action = Success

Choose one specific fitness goal and create a "WISH- DO- HAVE" equation.

"WISH" + "DO" = "HAVE"

"Wish" is your goal.

"Do" is your focused action.

"Have" is your positive result actualized.

Morning weigh in

Morning walk/jog/bike or Ashley's "Burn 'N Firm" – Total Fitness DVD

Breakfast or Mid-morning Meal

Coffee/tea/or personal choice

Blended smoothie with 1–2 scoops protein powder

OR:

Egg white omelet with salsa

6 oz. vegetable juice

Lunch

Roasted skinless turkey breast

Mixed salad with fat-free dressing, if needed, or steamed vegetables

Iced tea/natural low calorie soda

Afternoon Snack

Protein smoothie

Evening exercise

Aerobics dance class/elliptical trainer/treadmill/bike; plus 20 minutes of toning

Evening weigh in

Dinner

Grilled halibut

Steamed vegetables

Caffeine-free soda/iced tea/water

Evening Snack – optional

Baked/toasted tortilla and salsa

Day Seventeen

Dance like nobody's watching.

Action Step

Congratulate yourself each day knowing that you're not only increasing your aerobic capacity, you are also improving your dancing skills. Pride yourself on the fact that you're developing a new a new talent and building hand/eye and foot/eye coordination.

Don't worry about whether you're doing the movements "right," just keep moving and have fun.

Morning weigh in

Morning walk/jog/bike or Ashley's "Burn 'N Firm" – Total Fitness DVD

Breakfast or Mid-morning Meal

Coffee/tea/or personal choice

Blended smoothie with 1–2 scoops protein powder

OR:

Scrambled egg whites with peppers and onions

6 oz. vegetable juice

Lunch

Lean steak

Steamed broccoli and cauliflower

Iced tea/natural low calorie soda

Afternoon Snack

Protein smoothie

Evening exercise

Aerobics dance class/elliptical trainer/treadmill/bike; plus 20 minutes of toning

Evening weigh in

Dinner

Grilled haddock

Steamed cauliflower

Caffeine-free soda/iced tea/water

Evening Snack – optional

Rolled turkey slices with/without mustard

Cherry tomatoes and cucumber slices with fat-free dressing dip, if desired

Day Eighteen

"Habit simplifies the movements required to achieve a given result, make them more accurate and diminish fatigue." – Ashleigh Brilliant

Action Step

Drink More Water

Are you drinking enough? If you feel thirsty, you are already dehydrated. Drink a glass of water with each meal and between each meal. Hydrate before, during, and after exercise. Substitute sparkling water for alcoholic drinks at social gatherings.

Body Benefits: Drinking more water results in weight loss.

Dehydration can slow your metabolism. Water is your body's principal chemical component, comprising, on average, 60 percent of your weight. Every system in your body depends on water. Water flushes toxins out of vital organs, carries nutrients to your cells, and provides a moist environment for ear, nose, and throat tissues.

Morning weigh in

Morning walk/jog/bike or Ashley's "Burn 'N Firm" – Total Fitness DVD

Breakfast or Mid-morning Meal

Coffee/tea/or personal choice

Blended smoothie with 1–2 scoops protein powder

OR:

Egg white omelet (see Day Eight)

1 slice whole wheat toast with 1 tsp. light butter (such as Smart Balance)

6 oz. vegetable juice

Lunch

Lean hamburger with mustard, lettuce, tomato, and onion, without the bun

Iced tea/natural low calorie soda

Afternoon Snack

Protein smoothie

Evening exercise

Aerobics dance class/elliptical trainer/treadmill/bike; plus 20 minutes of toning

Evening weigh in

Dinner

Baked skinless chicken breast

Steamed vegetables

Caffeine-free soda/iced tea/water

Evening Snack – optional

Baked/toasted tortilla and salsa

Day Nineteen

"Discipline is remembering what you want." – David Campbell

Action Step

It takes discipline to say no time and again to friends, family, and co-workers offering you unhealthy food or unhealthy choices. Work on creating an automatic response, something you will say when someone offers you something you don't want to eat or suggests an activity that takes you away from your healthy lifestyle.

Why does it seem that people close to you go out of their way to sabotage you?

Getting fit through diet and exercise takes discipline. When we create changes in our life, some of these changes may affect our family, friends, and even co-workers. If your family and friends are supportive of your healthy lifestyle, let them know how much you appreciate their positive reinforcement; but if they're not supportive, they actually may be uncomfortable with your plan and (unintentionally) sabotage it.

Morning weigh in

Morning walk/jog/bike or Ashley's "Burn 'N Firm" – Total Fitness DVD

Breakfast or Mid-morning Meal

Coffee/tea/or personal choice

Blended smoothie with 1–2 scoops protein powder

OR:

6–10 hardboiled egg whites

6 oz. vegetable juice

Lunch

Two-cheese (fat-free) skinless chicken breast tacos with salsa

Iced tea/natural low calorie soda

Afternoon Snack

Protein smoothie

Evening exercise

Aerobics dance class/elliptical trainer/treadmill/bike; plus 20 minutes of toning

Evening weigh in

Dinner

Skinless Cornish hen

Mixed salad with fat-free dressing, if needed

Caffeine-free soda/tea/water

Evening Snack – optional

Microwave oil-free popcorn

Raw vegetables (celery sticks, baby carrots, broccoli, etc.) with fat-free dressing dip, if desired

Day Twenty

"Sometimes the most urgent and vital thing you can possibly do is take a complete rest." – Ashleigh Brilliant

The latest research indicates a strong link between lack of sleep and increased weight, and this may be just as crucial to shedding excess pounds as diet and regular exercise.

Sleep deprivation lowers leptin, a blood protein that suppresses appetite and seems to affect how the brain senses when the body has had enough food. Sleep deprivation also raises levels of grehlin, a substance that makes people want to eat.

Insufficient sleep has been linked with increases in fat tissue in the body and a loss of muscle strength and muscle mass. Lack of sleep causes a decrease in bone density, particularly in women, which can lead to osteoporosis.

When we are tired, we crave more sugar, caffeine, and refined carbohydrates, all of which can cause us to put on extra weight. When we do not get adequate rest, our adrenal glands are stressed and our kidneys will retain fluid, and we usually will appear puffy. If we get enough sleep, our organs will function more effectively and we will look better and appear thinner.

Americans average only a little more than six hours of sleep a night. The average adult needs eight hours of sleep a night, which means approximately nine hours in bed. People who sleep less than that have a 45% greater risk of being overweight, and those who sleep less than four hours have a 75% chance of being overweight.

Dr. Philip Eichling, a sleep and weight-loss specialist at the University of Arizona, says, "One of my treatments is to tell them [his patients] they should move from six hours to seven hours of sleep. When they're less sleepy, they're less hungry."

Action Step

Get more sleep. If your "Dump Your Trainer" fitness program requires you to get up an hour earlier every day, make an adjustment and go to bed earlier each night. You can start by gradually increasing your sleep 15 minutes per night until you get at least seven hours of sleep.

Make sure to avoid caffeinated beverages later in the day which may make falling asleep more difficult.

Morning weigh in

Morning walk/jog/bike or Ashley's "Burn 'N Firm" – Total Fitness DVD

Breakfast or Mid-morning Meal

Coffee/tea/or personal choice

Blended smoothie with 1 –2 scoops protein powder

OR:

Salmon Scramble (see Day Eleven)

6 oz. vegetable juice

Lunch

Grilled skinless chicken breast

Steamed broccoli and cauliflower

Iced tea/natural low calorie soda

Afternoon Snack

Protein smoothie

Evening exercise

Aerobics dance class/elliptical trainer/treadmill/bike; plus 20 minutes of toning

Evening weigh in

Dinner

Broiled cod

Steamed vegetables

Caffeine-free soda/iced tea/water

Evening Snack – optional

Cherry tomatoes and cucumber slices with fat-free dressing dip, if desired

Day Twenty-One

"We are what we repeatedly do. Excellence then, is not an act, but a habit." –
Aristotle

Over the course of your program, exercise and healthy eating will become your normal habits!

Action Step

CELEBRATE YOUR SUCCESS!

Every time you drop five lbs., lose an inch, feel stronger during your workout session, or have more energy – celebrate! Do something you enjoy, and thank yourself for all of the big and small victories you achieve. You're getting healthier, stronger, and closer to reaching your goal.

ALWAYS REVISE, REASSESS, AND RECOMMIT

Look at your progress and goals, and ask yourself the following questions:

What activities am I not doing now that might help me reach my goal if I began to incorporate them into my daily life?

What obstacles still need to be overcome?

How much do I want to achieve the goal?

Is my motivation strong enough?

Are the benefits achieved worth the costs?

What is the measurable outcome?

How will I feel when I reach my desired weight and my desired level of fitness?

Third

KEEP TRACK

Do a weekly review to monitor your progress. Review the past week and create an action plan for the upcoming week. Keep up the good work, and keep thinking healthy thoughts!

Morning weigh in

Morning walk/jog/bike or Ashley's "Burn 'N Firm" – Total Fitness DVD

Breakfast or Mid-morning Meal

> Coffee/tea/or personal choice

> Blended smoothie with 1–2 scoops protein powder

> **OR:**

> 6–10 hardboiled egg whites

> 6 oz. vegetable juice

Lunch

> Two-cheese (fat-free) skinless chicken breast tacos with salsa

> Iced tea/natural low calorie soda

Afternoon Snack

> Protein smoothie

Evening exercise

Aerobics dance class/elliptical trainer/treadmill/bike; plus 20 minutes of toning

Evening weigh in

Dinner

> Skinless Cornish hen

Mixed salad with fat-free dressing, if needed

Caffeine-free soda/tea/water

Evening Snack – optional

Rolled turkey slices with/without mustard

Raw vegetables (celery sticks, baby carrots, broccoli, etc.) with fat-free dressing dip, if desired

Evaluation/Reassessment Point

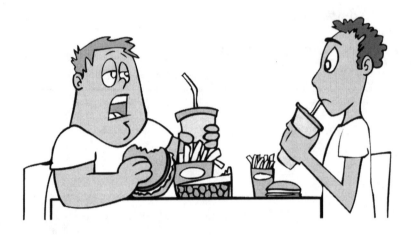

"Who needs a six-pack when I already have a keg?"

At this point, if you've kept to the program, you should have lost 5–15 lbs. From here, you have two choices. You can repeat the last 21-day program and continue to lose at the initial pace or greater, or you can modify the menu plan a bit and keep moving on, but at a more relaxed pace. If you're in Group #2 or higher, my suggestion is that you repeat the initial program until you're in the next lower group.

Some may want to substitute more lean chicken for the egg whites or lean red meat for some of the chicken. You may want to increase the amount of vegetables or add in a little more fruit. It's really up to you.

If you find yourself slipping back (the morning scale will tell you), then return to the start-up menu plan. But you must continue on the exercise program to really achieve your personal best.

If you haven't lost between 5–15 lbs., you need to take a critical look back at the last three weeks and acknowledge where you slacked off.

Remember the formula:

Calories expended MUST EXCEED calories consumed.

There is no way around this formula for the healthy person. If you didn't lose weight, then the inescapable fact is that you either cheated on your diet or you didn't get enough aerobic exercise to offset it.

Going to the gym and sitting around gabbing isn't exercise. Adhering to your diet and exercise program during the day and then pigging out on wine, cheese, and nuts at night isn't keeping to the program.

Only you know the answer, so only you know the solution. In any case, don't get discouraged. Making lifestyle adjustments is not as easy for some people as for others. Everyone has her /his own schedule and responsibilities, and changing one's lifestyle may be a more gradual process for some than for most. If you haven't seen the kind of improvement that you should have by now, it's very simple to reevaluate and begin again. Just consider, even a one-pound drop in weight per week can lead to a 52-pound loss over the course of a year. The most important point is to not get discouraged and give up. Go back, reevaluate, and acknowledge where you cheated. Adjust your mindset and try again.

From Here and Beyond

For those of you who have achieved Group #1 or who are moving along well in Group #2, there are some "sweeteners" you might want to add to your program which are not only fun and healthy, but downright addictive. One of these is Cardio Dance.

Cardio Lives!

If your goal is to improve your fitness level and lose weight, you must get cardiovascular exercise. PERIOD! There is no "best" cardio exercise. You can walk, jog, cycle, do Cardio Dance, or perform any other aerobic activity for at least 20 minutes. The many health benefits include:

- Helps control body weight

- Helps maintain and build healthy bones, joints, and muscles

- Improves mobility

- Promotes psychological well-being

- Reduces depression

- Reduces stress and anxiety

- Increases your lung capacity

- Reduce risk of heart attack, high cholesterol, high blood pressure, and diabetes

- Improves sleep

Warning! Don't listen to the "celebrity gurus" who advocate a cardio-free workout. Their absurd assertions include: "Cardiovascular exercise kills a weight-loss plan, your internal organs, your immune system, your time and your motivation..." (ABC News). This kind of gibberish may be appealing to those who want to avoid exercise and justify their unhealthy lifestyles, but the ultimate consequences could include diabetes, heart disease, osteoporosis, and more.

These gurus also neglect to point out that the key to sticking with your exercise program is making it fun! We challenge you to compare the exhilaration you feel during a cardio-intensive activity with the boring, tedious effort of trying to force yourself through an hour of an exclusively resistive routine. If you do, you'll quickly learn that these celebrity darlings are simply feeding you the misinformation they think you want to hear (so that you will buy their books). A year from now, they'll be telling you that the only exercise you need is lifting the fork to your mouth. Don't believe them! Again, *we didn't become a nation of fatties because of too much cardio.*

The truth is: You need cardiovascular exercise if you want to lose weight and reap the psychological and physiological benefits of a healthy, trim body.

If you live in a mild climate, take it outdoors – try hiking, walking, jogging, running, or cycling. If the city you live in is seasonally too hot or too cold to comfortably exercise outdoors, you can join a gym or a local recreation center. You'll have access to stationary bikes, elliptical trainers, treadmills, rowing machines, Stairmasters, and more.

Alternatively, home exercise programs can be ideal for some. Working out at home frees you of the commute, childcare fees, and any anxiety about working out in a group class or in front of others. Depending on your current fitness level and exercise preferences, there are numerous DVDs available in every fitness genre, including dance, kickboxing, step, and Tai Chi. If you want more information and reviews about fitness DVDs, you can visit Collage Video http://www.collagevideo.com.

Cardio Dance

I've been teaching fitness and dance programs for the past fifteen years. I've taught Bootcamp, Hip Hop, Step Aerobics, Kickboxing, Salsa, '80s Dance Party, Disco Divas, On The Ball, Circuit Training, Hi Lo, Ab Lab, Ballet Buns, and my signature series, "Burn 'N Firm." I learned firsthand that people make lasting changes when they associate happiness with exercise and feeling good. When we look at our lives and think about when we were most content, it's often when we were our healthiest. I've discovered that the key to long-term success is finding a program that you truly enjoy.

Dancing is a fun way to add variety to your cardio workouts. Not only are you burning a lot of calories, you're using every muscle in your body, improving coordination, and even improving your memory. As pointed out by Joe Verghese, M.D, et al, "Leisure Activities and the Risk of Dementia in the Elderly," *The New England Journal of Medicine*: "the only physical activity to offer protection against dementia was frequent dancing." His study demonstrated that reading led to a 35% reduced risk of dementia. Bicycling and swimming had no effect whatsoever but the protective effects of dancing were impressive.

Some people shy away from dance, thinking "I'm not a dancer, I have two left feet." But Cardio Dance is not about becoming a prima ballerina or a Latin mambo king. This is dance for fun and fitness, not a competition.

Cardio Dance classes at the gym are generally one hour, mixed level, fun, and non-competitive. You'll begin the class with a warm up, learning a few basic steps, and gradually adding more steps to create different patterns or choreography. The music, energy, and camaraderie should make you feel comfortable, even if you miss a step. In contrast, a class taken at a traditional-style dance studio where the focus is more on dance technique than cardio may leave you frustrated and sweat-less. This is not to discourage you from joining one, but you should understand that they have essentially two different purposes.

Don't be intimidated by the group of sweaty, smiling hip-shakers in the Cardio Dance class. Teaching classes, I've often had the experience of a woman coming up to me after class, beaming, and telling me that she had been watching the class for weeks as she walked on the treadmill and didn't think she could do the moves, but was so excited and had had a great time – along with a great workout! I love to see people leave the gym feeling confident, healthy, and energized.

The group dynamic is also a great motivator. So, if you've never taken any group exercise classes, give it a try – you may get hooked on a very healthy addiction. My groups of regular "Burn 'N Firmers" come to class religiously, and many have developed wonderful friendships as a result of taking the class. It's more than exercise, it's a social support system, as well.

Here are a few tips if it's your first time:

- Get to class five minutes early and let the instructor know that you're new to class. Tell her/him if you have any prior injuries and ask for any modifications you may need.

- Make sure you have the right type of shoes and are wearing sportswear you can move in freely. Pants that are too tight, or forgetting to wear a good sports bra (women), can ruin the class. Usually, a cross-training shoe with good lateral/ankle support (not a jogging shoe) works well.

- Don't worry about the right, left arms up, down, turn around movements at first – the less you think about it, the easier it will be. The instructor may "cue" the move before they do it; just follow along and keep moving. If you feel lost, go back to the basic move and add on when you can.

Don't worry that anyone is watching you. Trust me, most likely they're not. Rest assured that they're totally into their own routine and oblivious to anyone else's. If they do notice you, they're probably impressed that you're trying. Remember, they were beginners once too.

Women and men of all ages have told me that the workouts fly by because of the fun moves and music, and that it's a program which creates results that last.

A useful technique for starting this or any other new venture is to accept the fact that you are a novice and are going to screw up. This way, you have no expectation of keeping up with or outperforming anyone else, and can just relax and learn. You'll be surprised at how fast you improve when you take the pressure off yourself.

Spinning can be a great addition to your workout routine. The beat is exhilarating, the instructors are stimulating, and the exercise is definitely cardio-active. Unfortunately, the deafening volume of the music in many of the classes is extremely harmful to the hair cells in your inner ear and can lead to permanent hearing loss. If you can find a class with an acceptable music volume or don't mind wearing ear plugs, definitely try it.

"Wii" Fitness

Did you know that playing some video games can burn more calories than a typical workout with a Personal Trainer?

Recently, Nintendo has been developing and expanding its line of gaming software and peripheral devices to include video games which, although not sufficient to offset a full cardio-aerobic program, certainly can act as an adjunct to one. Although not yet currently measured, it seems intuitively obvious that the activities (tennis, dance, and even some fitness routines) expend more calories than those expended in a typical Personal Trainer session, and include a substantial amount of general body toning, as well. In addition, they don't require the participation of a partner, trainer, or even a workout buddy.

If you can afford it, we encourage you to consider adding some of their fun and exciting games to your home workout component, and ask that you look for the forthcoming "Dump Your Trainer" fitness video game, currently in development.

"Normalizing" Your Life

This term is really a misnomer. A normal lifestyle is a healthy lifestyle, and what you've probably been doing up until now is really better termed abnormal. Perhaps a more appropriate term would be liberalizing your lifestyle.

At this point, you should be metabolizing at a rate that allows for greater flexibility and freedom with your diet than during the start-up phases. Eating out in restaurants, at barbecues, and even having pizza and/or ice cream occasionally is no problem. Your exercise program should easily accommodate these rewards. In fact, you may find that you can eat just about anything – so long as you continue to burn off those calories. Your scale will tell you. You might even be surprised to find that eating isn't really an issue anymore.

Congratulations! You've made it. You've achieved a healthy lifestyle and can forget about dieting, just so long as you maintain your exercise program and follow the Dump Your Trainer Long-term Continued Success Diet Plan.

Look in the mirror and smile. You look great and you've come a long way.

The Dump Your Trainer Long-term Success Plan

Now that you've achieve your goal, you can feel pretty good about yourself and your new look. Maintaining a rigorous diet is no longer necessary, as long as you continue your exercise program. Eating healthy is a habit that you should embrace for life.

The following section will provide you with healthy, tasty dishes, and should help you not only maintain your new look on the outside but keep you healthy and fit on the inside. Of course, should you find yourself slipping back and packing on a few extra pounds, just return to the Dump Your Trainer Start-up Program for a bit of a boost.

Eat Right and Stay Slim

Most Americans consume too many calories and not enough nutrients, according to the latest revision to the Dietary Guidelines for Americans. In January 2005, two federal agencies – the Department of Health and Human Services and the Department of Agriculture (USDA) – released the guidelines to help adults and children ages two and up live healthier lives.

Currently, the typical American diet is low in fruits, vegetables, and whole grains, and high in saturated fat, salt, and sugar. As a result, more Americans than ever are overweight, obese, and at increased risk for chronic diseases such as heart disease, high blood pressure, diabetes, and certain cancers.

Of course, old habits are hard to break, and the notion of change can seem overwhelming. But it can be done with planning and a gradual approach, says Dee Sandquist, a spokeswoman for the American Dietetic Association (ADA) and manager of nutrition and diabetes at the Southwest Washington Medical Center in Vancouver, Washington.

"Some people can improve eating habits on their own, while others need a registered dietitian to guide them through the process," Sandquist says. You should definitely consider consulting a dietitian if you have a health condition such as osteoporosis, high blood pressure, high cholesterol, or diabetes.

Sandquist says that many people she counsels have been accustomed to eating a certain way, and never thought about what they were actually putting in their bodies. "Someone may tell me they drink six cans of regular soda every day," she says. "When they find out there are about nine teaspoons of sugar in one can, it puts things in perspective. Then I work with the person to cut back to three cans a day, then to two and so on, and to start replacing some of the soda with healthier options."

Sandquist says that when people strive for more balance in their diets, they tend to enjoy mixing up their food choices. "A lot of times, they've been eating the same things over and over. So when they start trying new foods, they find out what they've been missing."

Barbara Schneeman, Ph.D., director of the Food and Drug Administration's Office of Nutritional Products, Labeling, and Dietary Supplements, encourages consumers to make smart food choices from every food group. "The Nutrition Facts label is an important tool that gives guidance for making these choices," she says. The label shows how high or low a food is in various nutrients.

Experts say that once you start using the label to compare products, you'll find there is flexibility in creating a balanced diet and enjoying a variety of foods in moderation. For example, you could eat a favorite food that's higher in fat for breakfast and have lower-fat foods for lunch and dinner. You could have a full-fat dip on a low-fat cracker. "What matters is how all the food works together," Sandquist says.

Older people are most likely to improve their eating habits, but nutrition is important for people of all ages, says Walter Willet, M.D., chairman of the nutrition department at the Harvard School of Public Health. "We know that when people have health problems or their friends become ill, these are strong motivators of change," says Willet. "The more serious the health condition, the more serious the change. We'd rather people made changes early and prevent health problems in the first place."

Here are some tips to keep your eating habits moving in the right direction.

Look at What You Eat Now
Look for healthier versions of what you like to eat. If you like luncheon meat sandwiches, try a reduced-fat version. If you like the convenience of frozen dinners, look for ones with lower sodium. If you love fast-food meals, try a salad as your side dish instead of french fries.

Use the Nutrition Facts Label
To make smart food choices quickly and easily, compare the Nutrition Facts labels on products. Look at the Percent Daily Value (%DV) column. The general rule of thumb is that 5 percent or less of the Daily Value is considered low and 20 percent or more is high.

Keep saturated fat, trans fat, cholesterol, and sodium low, while keeping fiber, potassium, iron, calcium, and vitamins A and C high. Be sure to look at the serving size and the number of servings per package. The serving size affects calories, amounts of each nutrient, and the percentage of Daily Value.

The %DV is based on a 2,000-calorie diet, but recommended calorie intake differs for individuals based on age, gender, and activity level. Some people need less than 2,000 calories a day. You can use the %DV as a frame of reference whether or not you consume more or less than 2,000 calories. The %DV makes it easy to compare the nutrients in each food product to see which ones are higher or lower. When comparing products, just make sure the serving sizes are similar, especially the weight (grams, milligrams, or ounces) of each product.

Control Portion Sizes

Understanding the serving size on the Nutrition Facts label is important for controlling portions, Someone may have a large bottled drink and assume it's only one serving. But if you look at the label, it's actually two servings. If you consume two servings of a product, you have to multiply all the numbers by two. When the servings go up, so do the calories, fat, sugar, and salt.

Try dishing out a smaller amount on your plate, or use smaller plates. If you put more food in front of you, you'll eat it because it's there. According to the ADA, an average serving size of meat looks like a deck of cards. An average serving size of pasta or rice is about the size of a tennis ball.

Here are some other ways to limit portions: Split a meal or dessert with a friend at a restaurant, get a doggie bag for half of your meal, get in the habit of having one helping, and ask for salad dressing, butter, and sauces on the side so you can control how much you use.

Control Calories and Get the Most Nutrients

"You want to stay within your daily calorie needs, especially if you're trying to lose weight," says Eric Hentges, Ph.D., director of the USDA Center for Nutrition Policy and Promotion. "But you also want to get the most nutrients out of the calories, which means picking nutritionally rich foods," he says. Children and adults should pay particular attention to getting adequate calcium, potassium, fiber, magnesium, and vitamins A, C, and E.

According to the Dietary Guidelines, there is room for what's known as a discretionary calorie allowance. This is for when people meet their recommended nutrient intake without using all their calories. Hentges compares the idea to a household budget. "You know you have to pay all the bills and then you can use the leftover money for other things," he says. "The discretionary calorie allowance gives you some flexibility to have foods and beverages with added fats and sugars, but you still want to make sure you're getting the nutrients you need." For example, a 2,000-calorie diet has about 250 discretionary calories, according to the Dietary Guidelines.

Know Your Fats

Fat provides flavor and makes you feel full. It also provides energy, and essential fatty acids for healthy skin, and helps the body absorb the fat-soluble vitamins A, D, E, and K. But fat also has nine calories per gram, compared to four calories per gram in carbohydrates and protein. If you eat too much fat every day, you may get more calories than your body needs, and too many calories can contribute to weight gain.

Too much saturated fat, trans fat, and cholesterol in the diet increases the risk of unhealthy blood cholesterol levels, which may increase the risk of heart disease.

"Consumers should lower all three, not just one or the other," says Schneeman. Saturated fat is found mainly in foods from animals. Major sources of saturated fats are cheese, beef, and milk. Trans fat results when manufacturers add hydrogen to vegetable oil to increase the food's shelf life and flavor. Trans fat can be found in vegetable shortenings, some margarines, crackers, cookies, and other snack foods. Cholesterol is a fat-like substance in foods from animal sources such as meat, poultry, egg yolks, milk, and milk products.

Most of your fats should come from polyunsaturated and monounsaturated fatty acids, such as those that occur in fish, nuts, soybean, corn, canola, olive, and other vegetable oils. This type of fat does not raise the risk of heart disease and may be beneficial when consumed in moderation.

Make Choices That Are Lean, Low-fat, or Fat-free

When buying meat, poultry, milk, or milk products, choose versions that are lean, low-fat, or fat-free. Choose lean meats like chicken without the skin, and lean beef or pork with the fat trimmed off.

If you frequently drink whole milk, switch to 1 percent milk or skim milk. Many people don't taste a difference. Some mix whole milk with lower-fat milk for a while so the taste buds can adjust. "This doesn't mean you can never eat or drink the full-fat versions," Schneeman says. "That's where the discretionary calories come in."

Other tips to reduce saturated fat include cooking with nonstick sprays and using olive, safflower, or canola oils instead of lard or butter. Eat more fish, which is usually lower in saturated fat than meat. Bake, grill, and broil food instead of frying it because more fat is absorbed into the food when frying. You could also try more meatless entrees like veggie burgers, and add flavor to food with a low-fat bean spread instead of butter.

Focus on Fruit
The Dietary Guidelines recommend two cups of fruit per day at the 2,000-calorie reference diet. Fruit intake and recommended amounts of other food groups vary at different calorie levels. An example of two cups of fruit includes: one small banana, one large orange, and one-fourth cup of dried apricots or peaches.

Eat a variety of fruits – whether fresh, frozen, canned, or dried – rather than fruit juice for most of your fruit choices. "The whole fruit has more fiber, it's more filling, and it's naturally sweet," says Marilyn Tanner, a pediatric dietitian at the Washington University School of Medicine in St. Louis. Still, some juices, such as orange and prune, are a good source of potassium.

Ways to incorporate fruit in your diet include adding it to your cereal, eating it as a snack with low-fat yogurt or a low-fat dip, or making a fruit smoothie for dessert by mixing low-fat milk with fresh or frozen fruit such as strawberries or peaches. Also, your family is more likely to eat fruit if you put it out on the kitchen table.

Eat Your Veggies
The Dietary Guidelines recommend two and one-half cups of vegetables per day if you eat 2,000 calories each day.

Tanner suggests adding vegetables to foods such as meatloaf, lasagna, omelets, stir-fry dishes, and casseroles. Frozen chopped greens such as spinach, and peas, carrots, and corn are easy to add. Also, add dark leafy green lettuce to sandwiches. "Involve kids by letting them help pick vegetables in different colors when you're shopping," Tanner suggests. Get a variety of dark green vegetables such as broccoli, spinach, and greens; orange and deep yellow vegetables such as carrots, winter squash, and sweet potatoes; starchy vegetables like corn; legumes, such as dry beans, peas, chickpeas, pinto beans, kidney beans, and tofu; and other vegetables, such as tomatoes and onions.

"Look for ways to make it convenient," Tanner says. "You can buy salad in a bag. Or, buy a vegetable tray from the grocery store and put it in the refrigerator. Everything's already cut up and you can just reach in and eat it throughout the week."

Make Half Your Grains Whole

Like fruits and vegetables, whole grains are a good source of vitamins, minerals, and fiber. The Dietary Guidelines recommend at least three ounces of whole grains per day. One slice of bread, one cup of breakfast cereal, or one-half cup of cooked rice or pasta are each equivalent to about one ounce. Tanner suggests baked whole-grain corn tortilla chips or whole-grain cereal with low-fat milk as good snacks.

In general, at least half the grains you consume should come from whole grains. For many, but not all, whole grain products, the words "whole" or "whole grain" will appear before the grain ingredient's name. The whole grain must be the first ingredient listed in the ingredients list on the food package. The following are some whole grains: whole wheat, whole oats or oatmeal, whole-grain corn, popcorn, wild rice, brown rice, buckwheat, whole rye, bulgur or cracked wheat, whole-grain barley, and millet. Whole-grain foods cannot necessarily be identified by their color or by names such as brown bread, nine-grain bread, hearty grains bread, or mixed grain bread.

Lower Sodium and Increase Potassium

Higher salt intake is linked to higher blood pressure, which can raise the risk of stroke, heart disease, and kidney disease. The Dietary Guidelines recommend that people consume less than 2,300 milligrams of sodium per day (approximately one teaspoon of salt). There are other recommendations for certain populations that tend to be more sensitive to salt. For example, people with high blood pressure, blacks, and middle-aged and older adults should consume no more than 1,500 milligrams of sodium each day.

Most of the sodium people eat comes from processed foods. Use the Nutrition Facts label on food products: 5%DV or less for sodium means the food is low in sodium, and 20%DV or more means it's high. Compare similar products and choose the option with a lower amount of sodium. Most people won't notice a taste difference. Consistently consuming lower-salt products will help taste buds adapt, and you'll enjoy these foods as much or more than higher-salt options.

Prepare foods with little salt. The DASH (Dietary Approaches to Stop Hypertension) eating plan from the National Heart, Lung, and Blood Institute recommends giving flavor to food with herbs, spices, lemon, lime, vinegar, and salt-free seasoning blends.

Consult with your physician before using salt substitutes because their main ingredient, potassium chloride, can be harmful to some people with certain medical conditions.

Also, increase potassium-rich foods such as sweet potatoes, orange juice, bananas, spinach, winter squash, cantaloupe, and tomato puree. Potassium counteracts some of sodium's effect on blood pressure.

Limit Added Sugars

The Dietary Guidelines recommend choosing and preparing food and beverages with little added sugars. Added sugars are sugars and syrups added to foods and beverages in processing or preparation, not the naturally occurring sugars in fruits or milk. Major sources of added sugars in the American diet include regular soft drinks, candy, cake, cookies, pies, and fruit drinks. In the ingredients list on food products, sugar may be listed as brown sugar, corn syrup, glucose, sucrose, honey, or molasses. Be sure to check the sugar in low-fat and fat-free products, which sometimes contain a lot of sugar, Tanner says.

Instead of drinking regular soda and sugary fruit drinks, try natural low calorie soda, low-fat or fat-free milk, water, flavored water, or 100 percent fruit juice.

For snacks and desserts, try fruit. "People are often pleasantly surprised that fruit is great for satisfying a sweet tooth," Tanner says. "And if ice cream is calling your name, don't have it in the freezer. Make it harder to get by having to go out for it. Then it can be an occasional treat."

Smart Snacks

    Applesauce
    Low-fat yogurt with fruit
    Unbuttered and unsalted popcorn
    Broccoli, carrots, or cherry tomatoes with dip or low-fat yogurt
    Grapes
    Apple slices with peanut butter
    Raisins
    Nuts (a few)
    Graham crackers
    Gingersnap cookies

Low- or reduced-fat string cheese
Baked whole-grain tortilla chips with salsa
Whole-grain cereal with low-fat milk

Navigating the High-Fat Minefield

Okay, you've made the commitment to weight loss, fitness, and healthier living. Now, how do you stay with it when the world around you is committed to your failure?

Tips for Healthy Fast Food

- Look for items that are broiled or grilled; stay away from anything fried.

- Request extra tomato, onion, and lettuce.

- Ask for no cheese.

- Ask for no mayonnaise or "special" sauce.

- Ask for nonfat salad dressing or no dressing; use salsa if available.

- Look at the nutrition information to make the best fat gram or calorie choice.

Sounds easy, right? Wrong! Just try it. Decide that you're going to avoid that Big Mac and those fries. Tag along with your co-worker and head over to Burger King, KFC, etc., to pick up that salad. What do you think you'll really come back with?

As soon as you get within a block of that den of olfactory servitude, the smell of that fatty food is going to overcome you and – guaranteed – you'll be walking out with a double lard burger, jumbo fries, and shake. Sorry, but that's just the reality.

So, how do you deal with the overpowering urges passed on to you by your olfactory system? Well, the first thing you need to do is acknowledge the problem before you're confronted with it, and then try these simple suggestions from the doctor.

1) Don't go! That's right. Write down what you want and let your co-worker pick up that low-calorie, healthy lunch for you. Let them cave in to the temptation while you avoid it. One thing, though: when they bring back their jumbo fries, don't succumb to sharing them.

2) If you have to go, write down, in advance, exactly what you intend to order and have your friend order it for you. Or hand the paper to the counter attendant and let them execute it. Don't open your mouth to say a word. If you do, you're lost. Take your healthy order and walk/run away – quickly!

Unless you follow this advice devoutly, your new program is doomed to failure.

The following are some good choices. Make copies and have them available so you can just circle them when you hand them over.

Best Fast-Food Options

Subway
Order off the 6 Grams of Fat or less sub menu: lowest calorie sub is the Veggie De-lite, 230 calories, 2.5 grams fat, 37 grams carbohydrate, 7 grams protein Order off the 6 Grams of Fat or less salad menu: lowest calorie is the grilled chicken, 300 calories 3 grams of fat with fat-free Italian dressing

Baha Fresh

Mahi Mahi Ensalada
280 calories, 4 grams of fat, order with no cheese and use salsa for the dressing

Mahi Mahi Taco
177 calories, 9 grams of fat

El Pollo Loco

Flame-Broiled Skinless Chicken Breast
Order chicken skinless Calories: (155) Cholesterol: (95 mg) Fat: (4 g) Sodium: (540 mg) Exchanges: 4 Meat Protein: 29 g, Carbohydrate: 0 g, Fiber: 0 g

Pollo Choice Skinless Breast Meal
Order skinless chicken with fresh vegetables, garden salad & house salsa–use salsa as dressing, no tortilla Calories: (340) Cholesterol: (110 mg) Fat: (15 g) Sodium: Moderate (925 mg) Exchanges: 4 Meat, Bread, 2 Veg, 1 Fat Protein: 38 g, Carbohydrate: 16 g, Fiber: 6 g

BRC Burrito

Order with no rice,no cheese, add vegetables Calories: (375), Cholesterol: (15 mg) Fat: (14 g), Sodium: High (1255 mg) Exchanges: Meat, 4 Bread, 2 Fat Protein: 15 g, Carbohydrate: 60 g, Fiber: 6 g

Chicken Taco al Carbon

Calories: (135), Cholesterol: (30mg) Fat: (3 g), Sodium: (225 mg) Exchanges: 1 Meat, 1 Bread, Veg, Fat Protein: 9 g, Carbohydrate: 18 g, Fiber: 1 g

Sides

Steamed Fresh Vegetables Cal: 70, Fat: 4 g, Chol: 0, Sod: 80 mg, Prot: 3 g, Carb: 6 g, Fib: 4g Exch: 1 Veg, Fat

Pinto Beans Cal: 165, Fat: 4 g, Chol: 0, Sod: 715 mg, Prot: 8 g, Carb: 25 g, Fib: 10g Exch: Meat, 1 Br, Fat

Garden Salad Cal: 105, Fat: 7 g, Chol: 15, Sod: 135 mg, Prot: 5 g, Carb: 7 g, Fib: 1 g; Exch: Meat, Br, Veg, 1 Fat

McDonalds

Grilled Chicken Caesar Salad

100 calories, 2.5 grams fat, 3 grams carbohydrate, 17 grams protein, 1 vegetable exchange and 2 very lean meat exchanges. Choose one of the fat-free or reduced fat dressings.

Burger King

Chicken Whopper Jr.

344 calories, 14 grams fat, 31 grams carbohydrates, 23 grams protein. Exchanges: 3 starch, 2.75 meat (very lean). Without mayo: deduct 9 grams fat and 80 calories.

Whopper Jr.

order without mayo or cheese: 317 calories, 13 grams fat, 32 grams carbohydrate, 16 grams protein. Exchanges: 1.75 starch, 2 meat

Chicken Caesar Salad (no croutons)

220 calories, 5 grams carbohydrate, 7 grams fat, 3 grams fiber, 35 grams protein, no trans fat. With Italian Lite dressing, add 4 grams carbohydrate, 5 grams fat, 50 calories.

Side Garden Salad

25 calories, 5 grams carbohydrate, 2 grams fiber, 0 fat, 1 gram protein

Wendy's

Grilled Chicken Sandwich

300 calories, 8 grams fat, 36 grams carbohydrate, 24 grams protein. Exchanges: 2 starch, 3 very lean meat, 1/2 high-fat meat.

Small Chili

227 calories, 7 grams fat, 21 grams carbohydrate, 15 grams protein, 5 grams fiber. Exchanges: 2 starch, 1 high-fat meat, 1 very lean meat

Caesar Side Salad (no dressing or croutons)

70 calories, 4 grams fat, 2 grams carbohydrate, 7 grams protein, 45% Vitamin A, 30% Vitamin C. Use the Fat Free French dressing (80 calories, 19 grams carbohydrates, 0 fat) or one of the reduced fat dressings. For those on a low carb diet, the caesar dressing is the best option, it adds only 1 gram of carbohydrate, has 16 grams fat, 150 calories

Ordering At a Restaurant

Choose items that are prepared by low-fat methods – steamed, broiled, baked, grilled, stir-fried.

Eat a salad chock-full of vegetables without dressing with your meal – or better yet, order steamed vegetable so you can avoid the "fatty dressing challenge" altogether.

If you order a salad, ask for low-fat dressing on the side, or just add balsamic vinegar.

Skip the bread.

Grilled fish or chicken with steamed vegetables is a great choice.

Don't overeat! Use portion control!

You can check the nutritional value of almost everything at:
http://www.calorieking.com

"ALLI" – Oops!

Without going into great detail, let me just say that trying to lose weight through medicinal means such as stimulants, hormones, steroids, and the latest craze of (essentially) purgatives are doomed to failure.

 The distributor Glaxo-Smith-Kline, along with their compliant physician disciples, would have you believe that Alli is designed to be used by people who already have a low caloric intake of fat, to inhibit an additional percentage of fat from being absorbed, and thus, the side effects should be minimal. They advertise that people who are not able to limit their fat intake should not take Alli, due to its very unpleasant side effect of uncontrollable diarrhea.

 What a crock of… The fact is, people with low consumption of fat don't need Alli at all. What the manufactures don't tell you is that the real target consumers are actually the ones who can't limit their intake of fat and want a fast, simple, and artificial means of circumventing the issue. Of course, these are exactly the people who will have the highest incidence of the very unpleasant side effect (oops!), and shouldn't be taking the medication in the first place.

Unfortunately, people will probably have to learn this rather embarrassing lesson on their own. I just hope I'm not on the same trans-Atlantic flight as they are.

Dump the Car

Perhaps the single biggest culprit in the decline of our health and the expansion of our waistlines is the internal combustion engine. Prior to the invention of the automobile, if a person wanted to move something (including their fat asses) from one place to another, they had to provide the energy required to accomplish that goal. Today this is all done routinely by the car. Additional consequences, of course, include the heating up of our environment, the pollution of the air we breathe, and all the consequences that go along with it.

As portrayed in the cartoon below, one of the most pathetic anecdotes of our current lifestyle is the one about the gym member who lives within walking distance of the gym, but chooses to drive there anyway.

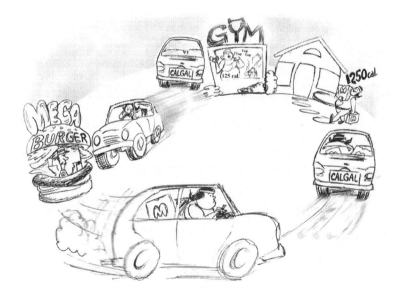

She searches diligently for the closest parking space, and then goes in and spends most of the one-hour "workout" with her trainer in minimal calorie-burning yapping about the congestion on the freeways or her poodle's heart disease. Of course, after the "workout," it's back in the car for a two-block trip over to Mega Burger. Total calories expended with her trainer: 125. Total calories consumed after such a "commendable" workout: upwards of 1250.

We've become a society addicted to our cars – and it shows. If you think I'm kidding, the next time you're at the mall, take a look around at the people there. The odds are pretty good that a large majority of them will be overweight, or even obese, and they won't be walking, they'll be waddling. That's what happens when you take walking out of your daily routine. You start to gain weight, and then you exercise even less. And since you continue to eat, the cycle gets worse as the weight gain intensifies.

For some reason, people seem obligated to drive everywhere these days. No one would ever think about walking more than a few blocks. That idea seems absurd; why walk when you can drive? But that is exactly the kind of mentality that is causing people of all ages, all across the country, to continue their love affair with the automobile.

You can burn an extra 300–1000 cal/day just walking. Driving to the store will burn about 50 calories. Walking will burn around 250. Same goes for all your little chores. Hey, no one is asking you to lug huge bags of groceries, but for small items, or those that fit in a cart, choose to walk instead of drive. The benefit will add up over time.

Sedentary Life Can Be Deadly

New studies are showing that a sedentary lifestyle can result in muscle loss and significantly lowered aerobic capacity.

Researchers at the Department of Physical Education at San Diego State University recently completed a 23-year study involving two groups of middle-aged men. One group exercised regularly for 23 years. The other exercised approximately five years and then stopped.

At the end of the study, when researchers tested the fitness of the men, they found those who hadn't exercised had lost 41 percent of their maximal aerobic power, while those who exercised lost only 13 percent. These results were interesting, since decreased aerobic power has long been thought to be a natural product of aging.

Additionally, the researchers found that none of the men in the exercise group developed high blood pressure, although two men in this group had high blood pressure initially. In contrast, 60 percent of the men who didn't exercise developed high blood pressure.

Another health bonus the researchers discovered was that the blood pressure of the men who exercised was 25 percent below the average for men their age.

The long-term health benefits from walking include:
Lower blood pressure. Exercise causes blood vessels to dilate, which reduces the pressure on blood vessel walls. Decreased pressure lowers the chance of a blood vessel rupturing in the brain, thus lowering the risk for a stroke.

Lower cholesterol. Exercise lowers your cholesterol level, which decreases the risk to your heart.

Strengthened heart and cardiovascular system. The elevated heart rate you get from walking will help lower your resting heart rate. A strengthened heart and cardiovascular system also lowers the risk of coronary disease and heart attack.

Increased bone density. As density increases, the risk of osteoporosis and bone fractures decreases. Weight-bearing exercise, such as walking, is especially important for women battling osteoporosis.

Production of growth hormones that counteract the effects of aging. As you grow older, your body stops producing hormones that help keep muscles strong. Therefore, regular exercise is the only natural way to get the body to continue to produce these hormones.

Increased production of endorphins. Endorphins improve mental and physical health, and are the body's natural way to decrease stress, helping you to relax. Forty minutes of walking three to four times a week can reduce depression and anxiety. As a result of endorphin release, people often find they feel better and sleep more soundly.

Weight loss or weight maintenance. Studies have shown that walking regularly can help you lose weight and keep unwanted pounds from returning. Depending on your pace, a one-mile walk burns approximately 100 calories for a person of average weight, and perhaps more for a heavier person (up to 300 calories per hour).

Strengthened nervous system and reflexes. When your body moves, the brain sends messages to muscles that tell the muscle how to work. Those messages must be passed frequently so that the nervous system continues to function, improving your reflexes.

Increased flexibility. Walking and stretching increase overall flexibility and make daily activities, such as climbing stairs, walking across the street, and driving a car, easier and safer.

Balanced insulin production. For diabetics, exercise increases the production of insulin, which helps combat the high blood sugar of diabetes. For non-diabetics, exercise may also prevent the onset of diabetes.

With such a long list of benefits, why not start walking more and driving less? You can do it; it's never too late to get started!

Health Tips

At least 10,000 steps a day for health – and more for fitness and weight loss. Each mile walked equals about 2,000 steps.

Allow 5–10 minutes at the beginning and end of walking to warm up and cool down.

Focus on the benefits and set realistic goals.

"Life Happens" Success Strategies

Here are my ten favorite long-term "Life Happens" success strategies that should help you maintain the progress you've made:

1) Eat Calorie-Balanced Meals

Spread your food intake evenly throughout the day. Keep track of your caloric intake. Work to distribute your total daily caloric intake between your meals and snacks. Aim to stay within the following calorie ranges:

- Breakfast: 300 to 500 calories

- Morning Snack: 100 to 200 calories

- Lunch: 400 to 600 calories

- Afternoon Snack: 100 to 200 calories

- Dinner: 350 to 550 calories

- Evening Snack: 50 to 150 calories

2) Schedule Your Meals

Think like an athlete in training. Food is your fuel! Avoid going long periods without eating. Plan your meals in advance.

For example:

  7:30 a.m. breakfast,

  10:30 a.m. snack,

  12:30 p.m. lunch,

  3 p.m. snack,

  6 p.m. dinner,

8 p.m. snack. (optional)

3) Eat a Healthy Breakfast

Start each day with a healthy breakfast that provides you with 300 to 500 calories. The Dump Your Trainer breakfasts will jumpstart your day and keep you satisfied. What you eat for breakfast is vital. Compare these two meal choices:

- o *Dump Your Trainer Breakfast:* Serving of oatmeal, 1/2 cup skim milk/soy milk, 2 slices turkey bacon or 2 links soy sausages/links, & 1 fruit with and a cup of tea or coffee contains only about 400 calories.

- o *Sugar Crash:* One pastry or muffin plus one cafe mocha drink is about 900 calories.

4) Snack Sensibly

Snacks are an essential part of your day. Plan ahead and carry small pre-portioned bags of almonds, (walnuts, or pecans), string cheese, fruit or cut vegetables. Snack mid-morning and mid-afternoon.

5) Be Mindful of Your Portions

Pay close attention to serving sizes. The portions we are commonly served in restaurants and even the food we prepare for ourselves is often too large.

- One fruit and vegetable serving is equal to one piece the size of a tennis ball.

- 3 ounces lean meat, chicken, or fish measures looks like a deck of cards.

- 1-ounce equals about 4 dice.

- 1/2-cup pasta or rice equals an ice cream scoop.

6) Drink Water

The Institute of Medicine advises that men drink about 13 cups of total beverages a day and women about 9 cups of total beverages a day. Make water your favorite beverage! Eliminate liquid calories (soda, juices, coffee drinks, sports drinks) from your day and drink water instead.

7) Live Alcohol Free

Remember you are "training" like an athlete; alcohol does not support your training. Save the calories and the headaches and say "no" to alcoholic drinks and "yes" to beverages that support your health and fitness goals.

8) Limit Eating Out/Make Good Menu Choices
By preparing all or most of your meals at home you can control what you're eating.

Eating out doesn't have to sabotage your healthy lifestyle. Try some of the following tactics to help make restaurant meals fit into your healthy eating plan

Tips for Dining Out: Get exactly what you want by being specific when you order, ask for healthy substitutions and:

- Choose restaurants that have healthy items on the menu.

- Avoid items prepared with cream or other heavy sauces.

- Hold the croutons, ranch and bleu cheese dressing– Salads are a great choice when you order your dressing on the side or ask for Balsamic Vinaigrette.

- Make a meal out of healthy sided dishes like: steamed vegetables, salad, chicken breast or black beans.

- Order meats that are grilled, broiled, roasted or baked.

- Order seafood that is broiled, baked, steamed, blackened, or poached.

9) Stop Eating 3 Hours Before You Go To Bed
By imposing an eating "cut off time" of 3 (or more) hours before bed, we automatically slash our calorie intake, commonly cutting 500 to 1,000 calories per day.

10) CREATE A NEW HABIT – 21-Day Transformation
A psychologically accepted length of time to form new habits is 21 days. The best way to get rid of an unwanted habit is to replace it with a good habit for 21 consecutive days.

- Keep a Workout Log

- Use Food Journaling

- Use the "21 Tips" included in the 21-Day Program to create healthy, positive motivation for fast, lasting results.

Breaking the Sugar Addiction!

According to the US Department of Agriculture, the average American consumes 43 teaspoons of sugar per day. The USDA recommends 10 teaspoons per day (less than what is in one can of soda). Sugar is often added to processed foods as; high fructose corn syrup, evaporated cane juice, cane sugar, fructose, barley malt or dextrose.

By reading labels, avoiding processed foods and changing our emotional eating habits we can break the sugar addiction.

Tips:

✓ If you are craving something sweet, eat fresh fruit.

✓ Only eat one serving of high quality dark chocolate and enjoy it.

✓ Don't buy tempting deserts. You will be less likely to eat it if it isn't in the cupboard.

I recommend using the herb Stevia as an alternative to sugar. It is 200 times sweeter than sugar and has no calories and unlike Artificial Sweeteners it is not a chemical. You can find Stevia at Whole Foods Market or your local health food store.

The Dump Your Trainer Real-life Meal Plan

Eating fewer calories while increasing activity is the best way to lose weight.

For most adult females, a diet of 1,200– 1,500 calories per day, and 1,500–1,800 calories per day for men is recommended for weight loss.

*Please visit http://health.ivillage.com/healthcalc to determine your target daily calorie intake.

Research shows that limiting calories, not the types of foods you eat, causes more weight loss. For example, cutting only carbohydrates or fats will not cause any more weight loss than a healthful and balanced low-calorie diet.

This meal plan has approximately 1200 calories per day, including snacks. This is suitable for most women (depending on level of activity). Males and more active females need to increase the total daily calories, adding up to 600 calories by increasing the portion size or adding additional snacks from the snack option list.

GOOD MORNING!

BREAKFAST OPTIONS: (coffee or tea is acceptable)

In the Mood for Eggs

Egg White Omelet

> 6 egg whites, lightly beaten
>
> 1 tsp. olive oil
>
> 1/2 cup chopped red pepper
>
> 1/2 cup diced zucchini
>
> 1 small tomato
>
> 3 sprigs fresh basil (or dry)
>
> 1 clove chopped garlic

Put olive oil in pan; add garlic, veggies, and basil. Cook over medium heat, stirring frequently. Add egg whites and scramble until cooked.

1 slice whole wheat toast with 1 tsp. light butter (such as Smart Balance)

Simple Eggs

Scrambled, poached, or hardboiled

2 pieces of lean turkey sausage or tofu sausage

Egg whites

1 serving oatmeal

1 cup skim milk or soy milk

Salmon Scramble

2 eggs or 6 egg whites

1 oz. smoked salmon, cut in thin strips

1 tsp. olive oil or spray

1 Tbsp. chives or other herbs to taste

Heat oil in nonstick pan over medium heat for 1 minute. Add eggs, salmon and herbs.

1 fruit serving

Omelet with Cheese, Please

6 egg whites

2 Tbsp. red and/or green bell pepper

1 Tbsp. scallions

2 Tbsp. reduced fat cheese

Spray nonstick cooking pan with cooking spray. Add pepper and scallions. Pour in egg whites. Add cheese. Fold.

Yogurt and Smoothie Options

Make sure the yogurt is nonfat/PLAIN or FAVE Greek nonfat yogurt.

Yogurt Crunch with Fruit

8 oz. or 1 cup nonfat yogurt

1/2 cup sliced fresh fruit (bananas, strawberries, blueberries)

1 Tbsp. flaxseed meal

3/4 cup low-fat cereal

Mix yogurt, fruit and cereal. *Add Stevia, if needed.

Smart Smoothie

8 oz. water

1 scoop/serving soy, whey, hemp, or egg white protein powder

1 Tbsp. flaxseed meal

1 tsp. psyllium husks

1/4 cup frozen or fresh blueberries

1/2 ripe or frozen banana, or other fruit that you like

Ice (optional)

Combine all ingredients in blender. Blend until rich and creamy, about 2 to 3 minutes.

Bitter Berry Smoothie

1/4 cup cranberries, fresh or frozen

1 cup blueberries, frozen

1 scoop/serving soy, whey, hemp, or egg white protein powder

1 Tbsp. flaxseeds

Combine all ingredients in blender. Blend until rich and creamy, about 2 to 3 minutes. *Add Stevia or other no calorie sweetener, if needed.

Super Sweet Smoothie

1/2 cup skim milk or soy milk

1/2 ripe banana

1/2 can crushed pineapple

1/2 cup nonfat yogurt

1/2 scoop/serving of soy, whey, hemp, or egg white protein powder

Combine all ingredients in blender. Blend until rich and creamy, about 2 to 3 minutes.

Cereal, the Breakfast of Champions

1 cup oatmeal

1/2 cup skim milk or soy milk

2 slices turkey bacon or 2 soy sausage links

1 fruit

OR

1 cup high-fiber/low-sugar cereal (e.g., Kashi, All Bran)

1 cup skim milk or soy milk

1/2 cup fruit

Don't Like Breakfast? You Gotta Eat Something

1 slice whole wheat toast

1 tsp. almond butter, peanut butter, or light butter (such as Smart Balance)

12 almonds

1 piece fruit

LUNCHTIME OPTIONS

Salad Lovers

Tuna Salad

6 oz. water-packed tuna, drained

2 slices tomato

1 cup romaine (or baby mixed greens)

1 cup cucumber and celery

Place salad ingredients in a bowl. Add 1/2 tsp. relish; mix tuna, mayo, and celery.

2 Tbsp. Fat free low sugar dressing

4 WASA crackers

Spinach Salad

1 cup fresh spinach

1 hardboiled egg

3 oz. sliced, grilled chicken breast

1 cup shredded vegetables

1/2 cup sliced mushrooms

2 Tbsp. low-fat dressing

Greek Salad

2 cups romaine

1/2 cup tomato

1/2 cup garbanzo beans

1 Tbsp. nonfat feta cheese (Trader Joe's)

1/2 cup cucumber

1/2 Tbsp. pine nuts

2 Tbsp. nonfat dressing

Grilled Hamburger Patty on Lettuce

1 extra lean hamburger patty

2 cups lettuce

2 Tbsp. nonfat dressing

1 cup vegetables

Tofu Salad

1/2 cup firm tofu, cubed

2 cups mixed green salad

1/2 cup vegetables

1 tsp. sesame seeds

2 Tbsp. nonfat dressing

Turkey Salad

3 oz. deli turkey

2 cups green salad

3/4 cup vegetables

1 Tbsp. Fat free, low sugar dressing

4 WASA crackers

Grilled or Baked Chicken Salad

3 oz. grilled or baked chicken

2 cups lettuce

1/2 cup vegetables

2 Tbsp. low-cal dressing

4 WASA crackers

Add 1 cup or 100-calorie serving of soup (low-sodium, low-fat brand) to any of the salad options.

Tuna Sandwich

2 slices whole wheat bread

1/2 cup water-packed tuna

1 tsp. reduced fat mayo

2 Tbsp. relish

Mustard

2 slices tomato

Ham or Turkey Sandwich

1 whole wheat pita

3 oz. lean ham or turkey

Mustard

1 Tbsp. reduced fat mayo

3 leaves of romaine

Bun-Free Burger

1 extra lean meat patty

2 oz. low-fat cheese

4 leaves green lettuce

1 Tbsp. reduced fat mayo

Mustard

Cook patty with cheese on top, place on lettuce.

Better BOCA Burger

Boca or veggie burger

1 toasted whole wheat bun

1 Tbsp. olive oil

2 slices tomato

3 leaves lettuce

1 slice red onion

Roll Ups

3 oz. sliced turkey, ham, chicken, or tofu

4 leaves lettuce

1/2 bell pepper, cut into strips

1 tsp. reduced fat mayo

1 Tbsp. mustard or reduced fat salad dressing

Place meat on lettuce, spread with mayo, and roll it up.

Need a Change from Sandwiches and Salads?

More Lunch Options

Chicken Kabob

4 oz. cooked chicken

1/2 cup green, red, or yellow bell pepper

5 cherry tomatoes

3 large mushrooms

Cut into pieces and put on skewer.

Taco

3 oz. lean ground beef, cooked and seasoned

1/4 cup cooked pinto beans

2 oz. grated low-fat cheese

Shredded lettuce

Tomato

1 corn tortilla, cooked with nonstick spray

Burrito

1 whole wheat tortilla

1/2 cup black beans

1/2 cup fresh or canned salsa

2 oz. low-fat cheese

Chicken Breast and Vegetables

4 oz. skinless boneless chicken breast, baked with seasoning

1 cup green beans or other vegetable

WINNING DINNER OPTIONS

Chicken Dishes

Chicken Pesto, Vegetables and Brown Rice

6 oz. boneless chicken breast (raw weight)

1 Tbsp. pesto sauce

1 oz. low-fat cheese

Cut slits in the chicken and coat with pesto sauce. Place chicken and sauce under hot broiler, cook for 6 minutes (3 on each side). Top chicken with cheese and place under broiler until cheese melts.

1/2 cup brown rice or small baked potato

1 cup steamed vegetables

Broiled Chicken Breast, Lentils & Vegetables

5 oz. skinless boneless chicken breast

1/2 cup cooked lentils

1 cup fresh broccoli

1 cup fresh or frozen green beans

Spray the chicken with cooking spray and broil until tender. Serve with the cooked lentils and steamed or microwaved vegetables.

Lemon Chicken Breast

1 skinless boneless chicken thigh

Lemon juice

1/2 Tbsp. olive oil

1 shallot

1/2 Tbsp. capers

1 Tbsp. Dijon mustard

1 cup steamed vegetables

Combine lemon juice, olive oil, shallot, capers and Dijon mustard for a marinade. Place chicken in shallow roasting pan and cover with the sauce. Broil for 12–15 minutes until chicken is fully cooked.

Healthy Chicken Fingers & Vegetables

4 oz. chicken breast tenders

1 tsp. chili powder

1 tsp. ground cumin

1/4 tsp. salt

1 cup steamed vegetables

Combine chili powder, cumin, and salt; rub spice mixture onto chicken. Place chicken in a baking pan coated with cooking spray. Cook chicken in preheated oven at 350° F, 15 minutes, turning every 5 minutes. Serve with low-sugar BBQ sauce.

Healthy Fried Chicken

4 5-ounce chicken thighs, skinned

3/4 cup chicken broth

1 Tbsp. olive oil

1 cup toasted wheat germ

1 tsp. dried tarragon

1 tsp. dried rosemary, crushed

1 tsp. fresh parsley, chopped

1 tsp. garlic powder

Salt to taste

Preheat oven to 350° F. Pour chicken broth and olive oil in a small bowl. In another bowl, mix together the wheat germ, tarragon, rosemary, parsley, garlic powder, and salt. Dip the thighs, one at a time, in the broth-oil mixture, then coat with the wheat germ and herb mixture. Bake in oven until brown and cooked through, about 45–55 minutes.

Beef Dishes

Garlic Steak and Potato

6 oz. lean filet or sirloin steak

1 tsp. olive oil

3 cup cooked green beans

1/2 medium baked sweet potato or baked potato

For the Garlic Butter

1 oz. butter

1 clove crushed garlic

1 tsp. chopped fresh parsley

Black pepper

Brush the steak with the oil on sides, then grill or barbecue to taste. Put the butter in a small bowl and mix with the garlic, parsley, and pepper. Serve over cooked steak. Serve with cooked green beans and sweet potato.

1 cup steamed broccoli

Beef Tenderloin and Mashed Cauliflower

4 oz. grilled beef tenderloin

1 cup mixed salad greens

2 Tbsp. low-cal dressing

Mashed Cauliflower

1 medium head cauliflower, cut into florets

1 cup purified water

2 garlic cloves, minced

1 tsp. fresh chives, chopped

1/2 tsp. onion powder

1/2 tsp. fresh parsley, chopped

1 Tbsp. chicken or beef broth

In a medium pot, place cauliflower in water and bring to a quick boil. Lower heat to simmer and cover. Cook for an additional 12 minutes or until soft. Drain, transfer cauliflower to a bowl, and mash. Blend garlic, chives, onion powder, parsley, and broth with the mashed cauliflower. Serve hot.

London Broil with Mushrooms (4 servings)

1-1/2 lb. London broil, 1-inch thick

2 tsp. dried rosemary

4 cloves garlic, minced

2 Tbsp. extra virgin olive oil

1 cup sliced white mushrooms

Rub half the garlic and rosemary on each side of the meat. Heat olive oil in nonstick skillet over medium heat. Add steak; cook for 5 minutes on each side. Transfer meat to another plate. Add remaining ingredients; cook for about 4 minutes. Serve with salad.

1 cup mixed salad greens

2 Tbsp. low-cal dressing

Fish

Salmon Teriyaki & Vegetables

Teriyaki sauce (makes enough sauce for 2 servings)

1/4 cup reduced sodium tamari sauce

1/4 cup dry sherry

1 Tbsp. sesame oil

1 Tbsp. grated fresh ginger root

2 garlic cloves put through a garlic press

1 salmon fillet

Combine the ingredients for the marinade. Place the fish in a glass or ceramic dish, pour marinade over it, and marinate in the refrigerator for 2 hours. Preheat the broiler. Remove the fish from the marinade and transfer to a plate. Grill the fish, basting with the marinade, for 3–4 minutes. Turn and grill, basting again, for another 3–4 minutes. Do not overcook. Serve with salad or steamed vegetables. (Low-fat dressing 2 Tbsp.)

Ginger Salmon

4 oz. skinless salmon fillet

1/2 clove garlic

1/2 Tbsp. grated fresh ginger root

1 Tbsp. low-sodium soy sauce

1 green onion

Place salmon in shallow dish, pour marinade over fish. Bake at 350° F until fish flakes, 20–30 minutes, basting with pan juices. Serve with fresh steamed broccoli.

Trout

4 oz. whole trout

2 garlic cloves

Fresh or dried rosemary

1 lemon

Salt

Pepper

Season fish with salt and pepper; place rosemary, garlic, and lemon on fish. Broil for 5 minutes, turn, broil 5 minutes, until fish is cooked through. Serve with steamed vegetables.

Quick Fish Dish

4 oz. fish fillets

1 clove garlic, minced

Fresh mushroom caps

Chives

Parsley

2 Tbsp. Italian low-cal dressing

1 tsp. lemon juice

Cherry tomatoes or quartered tomatoes

Lightly oil shallow dish or spray with cooking spray. Place fish fillets in single layer. Mix dressing with garlic and lemon juice, pour over fish. Sprinkle with chives and parsley. Dip mushrooms and tomatoes in dressing and put in pan around fish. Bake at 350° F until fish flakes, 20–30 minutes, basting with pan juices. Serve with fresh steamed broccoli.

Tofu-Vegetable Stir-Fry

1 oz. extra-firm tofu, cubed

1 cup vegetables (bell peppers, mushrooms, onion, broccoli)

1/2 tsp. toasted sesame oil

Cooking spray

1 garlic clove

1/4 Tbsp. red pepper flakes

Spray wok or nonstick skillet with cooking spray. Add sesame oil and sauté red pepper flakes on medium-high heat; add garlic, onion, and vegetables. Cook for 2–3 minutes, add tofu and stir-fry until heated through.

Thai Tofu Stir-Fry

1 oz. extra-firm tofu, cubed

1/4 can light (no sugar added) coconut milk

1 clove garlic

1 cup vegetables (bok choy, celery, bell pepper, asparagus, mushrooms)

1/4 tsp. red pepper flakes

1 tsp. light soy sauce

1/2 Tbsp. lime juice

Fresh or dried basil to taste

Mix coconut milk, garlic, and lime juice in wok, heat on high. Add vegetables, cook for 10 minutes or until vegetables are cooked as desired. Add tofu and stir in soy sauce and basil.

SNACK TIME

Choose two snacks per day from list.

Snack Suggestion List:

1 serving fruit
1 serving string cheese
1 Tbsp. peanut butter with celery
1 Tbsp. peanut butter with one small apple
1 serving sugar-free Jell-O
1/2 oz. raw nuts
1 oz. roast turkey wrapped round celery or carrot sticks
3 oz. fresh tuna with 2 cups of lettuce
1/2 cup low-fat cottage cheese or yogurt
Cut-up veggies

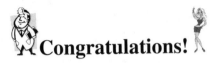

Congratulations!

If you've stuck with the plan you should have reached your goal! You've done it! Celebrate your success! Take a few moments to think about the changes that have taken place with your body and health. Write down all of the things that have improved for you since you started the Dump Your Trainer Program.

- Do you have more energy?

- How many pounds and inches have you lost?

- Are you stronger?

- Are you eating healthier?

- Has the way you look at your health changed?

- How have other areas of your life changed as your fitness changed?

Use this list as a reminder of your commitment to a healthy lifestyle. If you need extra motivation, keep a "before" photo as a reminder of all that you have accomplished.

Keeping the weight off permanently takes a daily commitment to leading a healthy lifestyle. Studies indicate that exercise is one of the most important things you can do for weight maintenance. To maintain your weight, use the tools that worked for you as you lost the weight: eating healthy meals and snacks, eating low-calorie, nutrient-dense foods, weighing yourself weekly to detect small weight gains before they become larger, using a journal to help you recognize any setbacks and to stay in control of your eating and exercise habits.

Continue to move forward and focus on all the wonderful benefits of your healthy lifestyle. Continue to share your success stories with us and inspire others to join the program.

Stay in touch at www.DumpYourTrainer.com

Appendices – Easy copy forms

1. Preparing for the 21-Day Dump Your Trainer Diet & Fitness Program – Strategic Plan

2. Personal Success Contract

3. Train Like An Athlete Action Foods

4. Sample Shopping List

5. Fitness Check Sheet – Evening Program

Preparing for the 21-Day Dump Your Trainer Diet & Fitness Program

Strategic Plan

"People with goals succeed because they know where they are going." - Earl Nightingale

The first step in making a real commitment is your belief in yourself; "I am doing this," instead of "I'm going to try to do it." The language you use is just as important as your physical actions. Create an inner and outer dialogue that is focused on the results you want. Know that you have the power to change your behavior and create the outcome you desire.

Take a few minutes to answer the following questions writing down the first three answers that come to mind:

Why do you want to change your body?

1.

2.

3.

What is preventing you from achieving your goal?

1.

2.

3.

Personal Success Contract

I, _____, commit to starting my fitness program today,

_____.

I commit to using the Dump Your Trainer – Change Your Life Workout Program consistently and following the Dump Your Trainer healthful eating program that will help me attain my fitness and health goals.

I will only fuel my body with the most nutritious foods possible.

I will be kind to myself and appreciate all that my body does for me.

I will strive to challenge my body and my mind.

I will acknowledge and reward myself for my achievements along the way.

_____

Signature

Sample Shopping List

Fresh Vegetables

Lettuce
Other Greens
Cucumbers
Carrots
Asparagus
Zucchini
Radishes
Tomatoes
Green Beans
Onions
Green Onions
Peppers
Cauliflower
Broccoli
Peas
Celery
Potatoes
Corn
Sweet Potatoes
Squash
Other Vegetables:

_____

_____

_____

Fresh Fruits

Bananas

Apples

Oranges

Pears

Peaches

Nectarines

Grapefruit

Berries

Other Fruits:

_____

_____

_____

Frozen Foods

Green Beans

Mixed Vegetables

Chicken Breasts

Fruit Juice Bars

Blueberries

Corn

Fish Fillets

Onions

Vegetarian Burgers

Other Frozen Foods

_____

_____

_____

Canned Foods

Black Beans

Tomatoes

Marinara Sauce

Tuna

Salmon

Pinto Beans

White Beans

Pineapple

Other Canned Foods:

_____

_____

_____

Meats

Lean Hamburger

Steaks

Fish

Shellfish

Chicken

Turkey

Ham

Other Meats:

_____

_____

_____

Grains and Cereals

Whole Grain Bread

Whole Grain Cereal

Oatmeal

Whole Wheat or Fat-Free
Tortillas

Other Grains:

_____

_____

_____

Beverages

Water

Coffee

Herb Tea

Other Beverages:

_____

_____

_____

Dairy and Eggs

Low-Fat/Nonfat Sour Cream

Low-Fat/Nonfat Milk

Egg Whites

String Cheese

Low-Fat Cream Cheese

L/N Yogurt

Other Dairy:

_____

Miscellaneous Items

Herbs and Spices

Low-Fat Dressings

Mustard

Almonds

Jell-O

Peanut Butter

Pecans

Olive Oil

Garlic

Popcorn

Salsa

Other Miscellaneous Items:

_____

_____

_____

Fitness Check Sheet – Evening Program

Aerobics

Arrive at the gym and begin with a five-minute warm up on either a bicycle or elliptical, if available.

Move over to a treadmill and make sure you again stretch out those gastrocs, etc.

Begin the step up component as in the morning exercise, and increase you pace in increments until you're jogging at 4.0–4.5 miles per hour (or greater, depending on your progress) for five-minute segments again.

Begin the step down sequence and decrease your pace at the same rate as the morning program.

Stretch out a bit. Congratulations! The aerobic component is done.

Toning

Exercise	Reps	Weight	Exercise	Reps	Weight
Floor or slant board crunches			Rotational weighted abdominals		
Overhead press machine			Angled forward press		
Biceps curls			Upper back pulls (row)		
Deltoid lifts			Lumbar (lower) back extensions		
Crunch machine			Gastrocnemius (lower leg) lifts		
Pectoral flies			Gluteus (leg) presses		
Forward press			Quadriceps (leg) extensions		
Full extension fly machine			Hamstring (leg) curls		
Backward fly's			Leg abductions		
Overhead pull			Leg adductions		
Free weight curls					

References and Resources

Consumer Reports, "Dangerous Supplements Still at Large," 5/2004. Consumers Union Publications.

Consumer Reports, "Comparisons of Diets," 2006.

The Musculoskeletal Manual, Bernbaum.

American Journal of Clinical Nutrition: "Physical activity and weight loss: does prescribing higher physical activity improve outcome?" October 2003. Jeffery, Wing, Sherwood and Tate.

Medicine & Science in Sports & Exercise: "Influence of exercise training on physiological and performance changes with weight loss in men." Kraemer, et al.

"Psycho-Cyb The Spread of Obesity in a Large Social Network over 32 Years." Nicholas A. Christakis, M.D., Ph.D., M.P.H., and James H. Fowler, Ph.D. ernetics, Dr Maxwell Maltz. *The New England Journal of Medicine*, July 26, 2007.

Williams MA, Haskell WL, Ades PA, et al. "Resistance exercise in individuals with and without cardiovascular disease": 2007. *Circulation* 2007; DOI: 10.1161/CIRCULATION AHA.107.185214. Available at: http://www.circulationaha.org.

US Department of Health and Human Services. "Physical Activity and Health: A Report of the Surgeon General." Atlanta, Georgia: US Department of Health and Human Services, Centers for Disease Control and Prevention, National Center for Chronic Disease Prevention and Health Promotion; 1996.

"American College of Sports Medicine Position Stand: the recommended quantity and quality of exercise for developing and maintaining cardiorespiratory and muscular fitness and flexibility in healthy adults." *Med Sci Sports Exerc.* 1998; 30: 975–991.

"Leisure Activities and the Risk of Dementia in the Elderly." *New England Journal of Medicine.* Joe Verghese, M.D., Richard B. Lipton, M.D., Mindy J. Katz, M.P.H.,

Charles B. Hall, Ph.D., Carol A. Derby, Ph.D., Gail Kuslansky, Ph.D., Anne F. Ambrose, M.D., Martin Sliwinski, Ph.D., and Herman Buschke, M.D.

"How to Keep Your Aging Brain Fit: Aerobics," *The Wall Street Journal*, by Sharon Begley, November 16, 2006

Index

228